Wade takes us on a transformational journey into the self, from the external and physical to the subtle, energetic, emotional, mental, and blissful bodies that make up who we are.

—Sharon Gannon, yoga teacher and cofounder of Jivamukti Yoga

Wade Imre Morissette offers a unique and practical approach to the koshas. He explores yoga not only as a physical practice, but as an experience of subtle energy and awareness.

—Yogi Vishvketu, Ph.D., founder of World Conscious Yoga Family and Anand Prakash Yoga Ashram in Rishikesh, India

Morissette's energy occupies every word of the book, and readers will feel deeply connected to his spirit. He provides inspiring teachings through his work and teaches out of his experience, rather than mere intellectual knowledge. I am sure this work will serve as a great inspiration for others in their own personal journey of transformation.

—Kausthub Desikachar, yoga teacher and yoga therapist at Krishnamacharya Healing and Yoga Foundation

Transformative Yoga

FIVE KEYS TO UNLOCKING INNER BLISS

Wade Imre Morissette

Foreword by Alanis Morissette

New Harbinger Publications, Inc.

Distributed in Canada by Raincoast Books

Copyright © 2009 by Wade Imre Morissette
        New Harbinger Publications, Inc.
        5674 Shattuck Avenue
        Oakland, CA 94609
        www.newharbinger.com

Cover design by Amy Shoup
Cover photo by Martin Prihoda
Interior yoga posture photos @Jaime Kowal
Text design by Amy Shoup and Michele Waters-Kermes
Acquired by Jess O'Brien
Written by Amanda Vogel
Edited by Jasmine Star

FSC
Mixed Sources
Product group from well-managed
forests and other controlled sources
Cert no. SW-COC-002283
www.fsc.org
© 1996 Forest Stewardship Council

Library of Congress Cataloging-in-Publication Data

Morissette, Wade Imre.
  Transformative yoga : five keys to unlocking inner bliss / Wade Imre Morissette.
    p. cm.
  ISBN-13: 978-1-57224-620-1 (pbk. : alk. paper)
  ISBN-10: 1-57224-620-0 (pbk. : alk. paper) 1. Yoga. I. Title.
  B132.Y6M69 2009
  181'.45--dc22

                 2009023485

11   10   09

10 9 8 7 6 5 4 3 2 1

First printing

CONTENTS

ACKNOWLEDGMENTS

There are so many people I wish to thank for support and assistance during the process of writing this book, most of all my family and my two beautiful boys for your patience and support during the last two years. I also extend a special thanks to my writer, Amanda Vogel of Active Voice Writing Service.

For assistance in production of this book, thanks go to Jess O'Brien and Jess Beebe for your amazing support; to everyone at New Harbinger Publications for making this book possible; to Jasmine Star for your skilled edit; to Dario Randi for creating the illustrations used in this book; and to Jaime Kowal for the yoga posture photography.

For other support along my path with yoga, thanks to Elana Maggal and and Renee LaRose from *Yoga Journal*'s conferences; to Terry McBride, John Rummen, and Dhyana Tse from Nettwerk/ Nutone Music; to Dave Waplington and Holly Gray for photo support and website maintenance; to Corwin Hiebert from Red Wagon Management; and especially to all my teachers in both India and North America for leading me through this journey of yoga. I send an extra measure of gratitude to my sister Alanis and to Alexi Murdoch for your inspirational music, which played in my ears while writing this book.

FOREWORD

As I write this, I am sitting in my office, listening to Wade Imre Morissette's song "Ganapati," and reflecting on how radically I have been influenced by Wade, my twin brother. Throwing any concerns of bias out the window (what is bias, really, other than an assessment based on knowing someone?), I begin reflecting on how I can possibly distill my thoughts around how I feel about this book, and about the man himself.

I am deeply struck by how Wade has supported me at countless junctures throughout my life—most recently, by way of his music and yoga teaching. Whether through his encouragement, his unwavering and sharp humor, his humility, his aliveness, or his fascination with bridging aspects of humanity and divinity, he has shown a visionary and steadfast commitment to truth and to removing any obstacle that keeps the people he cares for from discovering the highest truth about themselves.

At some times, his example has shaken me; at other times, it has inspired me; at other times, it has uplifted me. I notice shifts in my cells from every interaction with Wade, whether it's his soothing kirtan music and performances, his tenacious inquiries, or his yoga instructions in his classes. His compassion is unwavering, and he has an uncanny ability to bring levity and insight to any subject, whether mundane or profound. As he has entered the more formal yogic realms over the last two decades, his service has become even more distilled and focused. When I learned he was writing a book, I clapped my hands together and said, "I'm so happy! Now everyone can get a glimpse of what has been so profoundly moving to me!"

The essence of my brother could never be contained in one record or one book. The totality of his contribution will be felt cumulatively over his lifetime, through his generous performances, the brilliant yoga teacher trainings and workshops he leads worldwide, his casual yet consistently empowering presence, and his art, his writings, and any other form of expression he chooses to entertain in the years to come.

That said, the book you hold in your hands offers great support and guidance to help you integrate aspects of spirit, emotion, intellect, ritual, tradition, discipline, and application. In a way that's practical and succinct, Wade will show you how to bring all the many aspects of life home to the blessed temple that is your body.

As a person who can get stuck in the cognitive, intellectual, and conceptual aspect of things, I find that the teachings and wisdom in this book serve as a great guide to me in entering what feels like an imperative frontier. On the one hand, the book speaks to the ways the body can serve as a barometer, indicator, and messenger. On the other hand, it speaks directly to honoring the body and caring for it in a way that will allow your strength, flexibility, awareness, and practice to permeate every aspect of your life.

I remember being at a workshop Wade was giving in New Zealand and quietly saying to myself that Wade has miraculously achieved a great feat: he knows and honors the span of the yogic traditions, and at the same time, he pushes the yogic envelope forward by being progressive, playful, practical, and certain.

May this book serve you and hold you on your journey, and may you be as moved and supported as I have been by Wade's knowledge, experience, and generosity.

—Alanis Morissette

INTRODUCTION

Yoga is more than five thousand years old, yet the science, spirituality, and system it embodies is as relevant today as when it was first developed, if not more so. The theory and practices in this book were born out of an ancient discipline but have been designed for twenty-first-century life, *your life*. The intention is to foster a deeper sense of happiness and peace in your day-to-day existence, whether you already practice yoga or you're coming to it for the first time with this book.

Although the yogic tradition derives from India, today's Western world has adopted yoga as a popular form of fitness practice, and for good reason. Yoga brings about psychosomatic changes in how we feel and relate to ourselves and others—physically, emotionally, mentally, and spirituality. Physically, yoga heals by strengthening and relaxing the body. Yoga postures increase flexibility, prevent and reduce symptoms of disease and injury, and release bodily tension. Yoga increases feelings of vitality and energy, in part by expanding your capacity to breathe deeply, which moves *prana* (your body's life force). Stagnant energy, or unmoving prana, can lead to disease and depression. On the other hand, the movement of prana generates vitality, a stronger immune system, and resilience to disease.

Yoga heals emotions, as well, by encouraging an emotional intelligence that helps with facing pain, sorrow, suffering, and loss. Yoga is truly transformative on every level.

Through yoga practice and contemplation, you learn to quiet your mind and focus your thoughts, two important strategies for living in our fast-paced, technologically advanced society. Even if you don't currently practice yoga, you may have noticed a time when being mentally calm and present versus stressed-out and distracted helped you better handle an everyday situation, such as pulling together a last-minute presentation at the office or dealing with a toddler's temper tantrum. However, the mental focus that yoga instills extends beyond this sort of minutiae of life. A calm mind leads to deeper experiences too, such as a greater trust in the flow of the universe, increased creativity, and a heightened power to move toward realizing your dreams for your life. Finally, whatever your religious orientation, yoga allows a reverence of spirit that provides a firm foundation for daily life and infuses it with joy. In essence, practicing yoga opens the door to creating a new state of being. And with this new state of being comes a new perspective, one that leads you back to wholeness—to your true self.

Consider for a moment that your thoughts and intentions can create your life. For most people, this notion is easier said (or, rather, thought) than put into action. That's because it helps to have a path, constructed of tangible stepping stones, to bring such a theory into real-world practice. This book is that path. It's a guide for bringing yourself more in alignment with your deeper, more meaningful layers of being.

In this book, you'll learn how to apply the yogic philosophy of *koshas* to your own circumstances and experiences. *Kosha* is a Sanskrit word meaning "layer" or "sheath." As you journey through this book, you'll uncover layers of yourself on a journey of personal discovery that will move progressively inward, from the familiar physical dimension (in the form of yoga poses) to a more refined, subtle, and deep sense of consciousness. Layer by layer, you will transcend toward your true essence using the practical steps in each chapter to help you unveil your own inner bliss. The effects are profound and long-lasting, as I discovered through my own experience.

MY STORY

My journey toward the healing effects of yoga began in 1993. At the time, I was seeking relief from emotional stress on both a conscious and an unconscious level. During my first year at college, I was a mess inside. I desperately lacked inner peace, although this wasn't outwardly apparent.

My parents had recently gone bankrupt, so I was exhausted from working three jobs between high school and college to pay my tuition, and I continued to work part-time while in college. The daily grind was unfulfilling, to say the least. Meanwhile, my twin sister, Alanis Morissette, exploded onto the music scene with her groundbreaking album *Jagged Little Pill*, which went on to become the highest-selling debut album of all time. With her rapidly mounting success, I felt more emotionally and spiritually lost than ever before and longed to find my own identity and path in life.

I was studying to become an environmental lawyer, a vocation I had an interest in, but one that didn't fully satisfy me. Deep down, I knew academic study wasn't going to fulfill my quest for inner peace and happiness. Most of the books I was required to read focused on theory. I needed truth—an unwavering, blatant truth with no smoke and mirrors. In the end, I decided not to complete a degree in environmental law. Ironically, though, the time I spent at college led me in a different and unexpected direction: toward a new sense of spirituality.

It was my university roommate—a hippie at heart studying to be a librarian—who had a hand in changing the course of my life. He suggested I read *The Mystic Path to Cosmic Power*, by Vernon Howard. The book's conversation about God and how to attain a connection to spirit interested me most. Could leading a more spiritually conscious life allow me to feel more peace, joy, and unconditional love? In search of the answer, I delved deeper into readings on Eastern mysticism and philosophy, often reading until five in the morning then sleeping late in the day. My peers thought I was crazy, and in a way, they were right—I was going crazy as I yearned for inner peace and mental composure. Through my exploration of all things pertaining to God and a higher power, I realized that I needed to adopt a daily spiritual discipline. I explored karate-do but didn't care for the sparring aspect of it. I tried Taoist tai chi, which I enjoyed, but found too gentle. At that time, I still didn't know about yoga.

After leaving college, I moved from eastern Canada to Vancouver, British Columbia. I was drawn to Vancouver's socially conscious community, but I also saw it as a geographical step closer to Asia, the home of all the spiritual readings I had pored over and the continent I hoped to visit someday. That dream became a reality after I began to feel a strong pull toward India. To this day, I can't explain why I was drawn there, except that it brought me closer to my life's calling: yoga.

I quit my job at a health food store and booked a flight to Chennai (formerly Madras). Once there, I hopped on a bus to Mahabalipuram. I vividly remember walking down the street in that small village and spotting a sign: "Hatha Yoga—Upstairs, 5:30 p.m." I went to the advertised class, and from then on I was hooked. I sampled as many yoga classes as I could during my travels around India.

I became a *sannyasin* (Sanskrit for "spiritual seeker") at a meditation center called Osho Ashram in Pune. In Varanasi, I meditated with *sadhus*, yogis dedicated to meditation and contemplation of God. Once, after we'd sat for hours in meditation, a sadhu said to me, "This is the real yoga." He meant yoga was more than doing a series of physical postures without mindfulness. I realized then that yoga is as vast as the ocean, and that meditation is the ultimate key to yogic transformation.

Since my initial introduction to yoga, I've studied with some of the world's greatest teachers and masters, in both India and the West. My practice continues to grow deeper and more diversified. And although I now train other yoga teachers, I still consider myself a student of yoga. It keeps me humble and open to learning.

My opportunity to learn from many enlightened yoga masters has taught me that there is no right or wrong way to practice yoga. Yoga isn't something you learn, and then you're finished. Yoga is a lifelong journey and commitment. And it doesn't matter what style of yoga you practice; there is no *one* way. The most important gauge for determining whether you're practicing yoga correctly is how you feel. If you feel better after practice, you're doing it right! On the other hand, if your practice makes you feel worse, that's a sign that something needs to be adjusted.

This book isn't about categorizing yoga into nice, neat boxes. It's about practicing yoga in the broad sense in which it was meant to be practiced. It's about cultivating a discipline that is ever-changing—adapting it to serve you wherever you find yourself—in space and time, and in body and spirit. Your practice should change as you change. The only constant is this: What you experience through yoga should feel good to you. And that's where the koshas—your keys to inner bliss—become especially important.

THE FIVE KOSHAS AND ATMAN

Despite several yoga-inspired trips to India and enlightenment lessons from various yoga masters, I first stumbled upon kosha theory in a more everyday way: at the local library. I was looking through the Upanishads—a large, ancient text from India—when I found a section describing the life-affirming qualities of the koshas. The kosha philosophy resonated with me because it provided a blueprint for personal fulfillment that applies as much today as it did thousands of years ago—something that can't be said of many other yogic philosophies. Simply put, the koshas set a foundation for whatever roles you play in modern life—parent, spouse, daughter, son, businessperson, employee, artist, teacher, or any number of other titles you use to describe yourself.

According to the theory, every person possesses five koshas, or layers of energy. For the purposes of this book, I call these layers physicality, energy, meditation, awareness, and profound inner peace. The outer layer resides in the physical dimension: what you can see, feel, and touch. This is the kosha you will focus on first. As you work through the chapters in order, moving deeper through your koshas, you will arrive at more subtle energy bodies as you draw your attention to your thoughts and emotions, personal awareness, inner joy, and, finally, deeper into the essence of your soul. Once you've transcended and purified each of the five layers through practices you'll learn in this book, you'll be able to move between the koshas with ease.

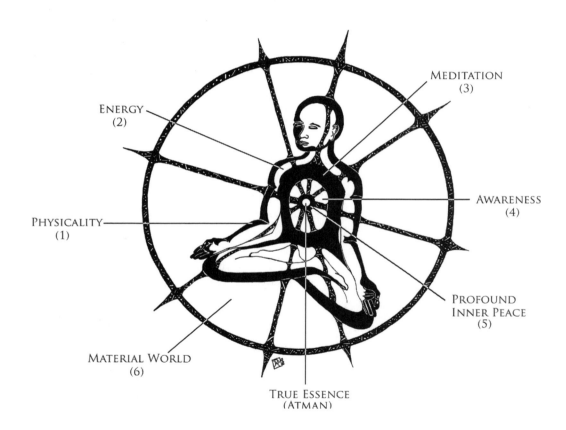

ENERGY
(2)

MEDITATION
(3)

PHYSICALITY
(1)

AWARENESS
(4)

PROFOUND
INNER PEACE
(5)

MATERIAL WORLD
(6)

TRUE ESSENCE
(ATMAN)

Each layer brings you closer to a deep sensitivity and awareness about yourself and your connection to spirit, and at the center of the five koshas is *Atman*, meaning your soul or true essence. Atman is God and truth. Of course, you can't live in the world of Atman all the time, but you can create a stronger tie or connection to Atman, similar to how a fetus is attached to its mother and nourished by an umbilical cord.

It's easy to forget your true self as you get caught up in day-to-day life. In ancient India, many yoga masters encouraged their devotees to leave common life for an existence of meditation and contemplation. That's hardly possible today. Imagine telling your family, friends, and coworkers you're dropping out of society in search of your Atman! You can't do that, and you probably don't want to, either. By following the modern kosha blueprint laid out in this book, you'll learn how you can live life as you need to—going to work, raising your kids, caring for others—but with greater fulfillment and joy.

CHAPTER 1

PHYSICALITY

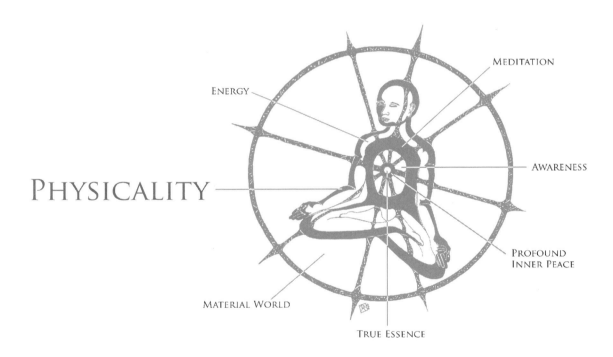

PHYSICALITY

ENERGY

MEDITATION

AWARENESS

PROFOUND INNER PEACE

MATERIAL WORLD

TRUE ESSENCE

When you first think of yoga, you probably imagine its most common feature: the physical practice. You may have observed a yoga class or spotted photos of yoga exercises in a magazine. You might even know what yoga feels like because you've experienced it a few times, or maybe you already practice it quite regularly. For most people, yoga begins at a physical level. And for some, it ends there too. This book delves deeper into the yogic experience, guiding you on a journey that will take you far beyond the physical. However, the path inward through the five koshas begins with your physicality, which is the first, outermost kosha.

Exploring physicality first is important because the body is the doorway to your more subtle layers of being. It's tricky to access the deeper kosha sheaths purely through meditation and deep introspection. The idea behind kosha philosophy is that once you clarify or purify each of the five layers, the glow of your true essence and inner bliss becomes more apparent.

The process of purifying each kosha doesn't change the kosha per se. Each kosha layer remains the same in its elements; it just takes on a purer quality. One way to illustrate this idea is to think about tainted water. Filtering the water purifies it, but it doesn't essentially change it—it remains water. The water's overall properties are the same, just purer. This is also true of the koshas.

Another way to illustrate the koshas is to think of your true essence as a lightbulb in a lamp; the kosha layers are like lampshades. Unhealthy koshas block your true essence from emitting a good amount of light. However, you don't take off the lampshades so the light can shine more brightly. You clarify the layers so they become more translucent, revealing the light within.

MINDFUL PHYSICALITY

If the body is full of toxins or in pain due to impurities in the physical kosha layer, it's difficult to concentrate fully on your inner self. Imagine trying to sit in peaceful meditation when you're distracted by impossibly tight muscles or buzzed out on caffeine. On a more serious note, when your body is fighting disease, you're more likely to experience difficulty accessing the deeper planes of consciousness.

While it's true that your body offers a direct link from the physical world to your deep consciousness, there are many distractions along the way. The advancement of technology combined with the speed at which we seem to live in today's world may distance and even disconnect you from your inner bliss. Engaging in yoga as a physical practice helps close that gap.

In fact, it's important to attend to the integrity of your physical practice because the center of consciousness is rooted in the physical—your spine and brain. Your spine is the pathway to a higher state of consciousness where you are more attuned to your true essence, or Atman. Energy flows through the spine to the brain, and if your spine isn't healthy, meaning mobile and supported by strong back musculature, the energy may be blocked. The brain is the site of the pineal gland, where the third eye is located. As conceptualized in yogic thought, the third eye is one of seven major chakras in the body. Chakras are energy vortices located along the spine. The third eye, or brow chakra, is known as the seat of consciousness. This very literal mind-body connection demonstrates how the gross, physical self is closely intertwined with more subtle layers of consciousness.

AN OUTWARD EXPRESSION OF YOUR INNER SELF

Consider also that your physicality is an outward expression of your inner self. Your external self—meaning how you appear to others—says a lot about your internal state. Everything from your facial expressions to how you hold your body tells a story about your inner life. Do you smile easily and often, or are you prone to frowning or scowling? Do you carry yourself with confidence? How do you stand and sit? Is it with good posture, or do you slouch? What about the energy you put out to the world? What does it say about the state of your inner bliss, or lack of it?

Think back to a time when being stressed about life's circumstances caused you to become ill, perhaps with an ordinary cold, a headache, or an ulcer, or maybe something more serious. It's difficult to hide your inner layers in the material world. This is true whether your inner self is in turmoil or in a healthy, blissful state. Of course, if you're experiencing deep bliss, your outer self will naturally show it; you will look more radiant and exude vitality. If, however, things aren't going so well in your inner world, you are bound to experience physical blockages, maybe in the form of disease, muscular tension, and pain. And guess what? The more you try to hide your internal state, the more it tends to manifest outward.

Now if you're hoping that a dedicated yoga practice will eventually rid you of stress, please back up and rethink that notion. Stress is part of being human, and it's very difficult, if not impossible, to be completely free from stress. You might feel pretty stress free while on vacation or during and immediately after your yoga practice. But it's hard to maintain that feeling all of the time. One hour, one day, or one week of relaxation isn't enough to reach a deeper level of awareness; it's your relationship to stress that makes the difference. How you handle and react to stress is the greatest indicator of your spiritual state. It's not about being perfect. It's not about escaping stress. It's about cultivating physical and emotional strength and releasing tension from both your body and mind.

Your yoga practice, and its stress-reduction benefits, will bring you energy. You'll feel this energy as you become familiar with practicing yoga postures. You'll also learn how to access the greater wisdom that lies within—a wisdom that's intimately connected to your own bliss and joy. But beware: This state of being doesn't arrive at a singular point in time. And it doesn't turn on and stay on indefinitely. Rather, feelings of joy will wax and wane, coming and going in cycles that repeat themselves from the beginning of your path to the end of your life. And so the journey begins.

THE POWER OF PHYSICALITY

As mentioned, the simplest gateway into yogic spiritual practice for most people is through the physical practice of yoga postures. You will probably find this physical practice the most accessible kosha to experience simply because you're used to moving your body, even if you don't currently exercise. You already know what it's like to live in the physical world, which makes the physical sheath easier to relate to than some of the deeper koshas. Starting on this familiar level sets you up for success as you journey toward a deeper awareness of yourself and your potential for inner bliss. Once you journey deeply into and ultimately transcend your physical body, it becomes easier to get in touch with the subtler aspects of your existence.

However, don't be fooled. The physical kosha may be the most familiar, but in many respects it's one of the hardest koshas to transcend. Believe it or not, your physical self requires the most work because it's your outer shield, your defense against disease, anxieties, and external stressors and

Historically, yoga was practiced by sadhus—renunciates who withdrew from common life to engage in self-inquiry about the fundamental nature of existence. As part of this quest for deeper meaning, sadhus observed animals and created yoga postures that physically mimicked them, developing what we now know as the animal-named poses, such as Downward Dog and Pigeon.

pollutants. The tensions in your body run quite deep. Plus, on a physical level, you're constantly immersed in the five senses—sight, sound, taste, touch, and smell—and it's very hard to withdraw from the senses. Luckily, once you penetrate this outer layer, you can move more quickly toward your deeper sensibilities.

MINDFUL NUTRITION FOR PHYSICAL PURIFICATION

Although the focus of this book isn't on nutrition, it's apropos to include a brief section here on the physical and even metaphysical benefits of mindful eating. Think of your dietary habits as an opportunity for bodily purification. In our modern world, there are far too many pollutants and toxins associated with the growth, production, distribution, and consumption of much of our food supply. Whether you're vegetarian, vegan, omnivorous, or subscribe to some other diet, your overall food choices play an integral role in the purification process.

The more you optimize your nutrition, the more easily you'll move through the koshas outlined in this book. Peak physical health fosters a transcendence to spirituality. To that end, the common aim for many yogis is to sustain a vegetarian diet. One reason is because of the many toxins found in cattle and other creatures bred for human consumption. Having said that, not everyone will pursue vegetarianism, for a wide range of reasons. If meat is part of your diet, select organic, free-range meat from grass-fed animals whenever possible. Opt for red meat less often and fish more often. When it comes to fruits and vegetables, it's also worthwhile to buy organic.

Perhaps most importantly, know yourself with regard to your diet. Select foods that support your energy requirements and make you feel physically good. And be sure to eat slowly. This will help you avoid overeating; plus, mindful eating produces happy digestion.

Here are some commonsense nutrition tips for cleansing and purifying your body to help you prepare for transcending to the deeper koshas through yoga.

Lighten up on sugar. Foods that are full of refined white sugar, high-fructose corn syrup, or even evaporated cane juice tend to create a short burst of energy followed by a longer low. When you plummet to that low, you may feel the need to consume more sugar or caffeine to energize yourself, which creates a counterproductive cycle of unhealthy nutrition. If you just can't quit eating sugar, at least try to cut down on it. For example, avoid adding sugar to items that may already be sweetened, such as breakfast cereal. And whatever you do, steer clear of artificial sweeteners as a way to avoid sugar.

Cut down on caffeine. How many times a day do you drop by your local java joint or brew up some coffee at home or at work? Not only does caffeine dehydrate the body, it can also make you feel downright jittery, which interferes with your ability to turn your focus inward and enjoy a calming yoga practice. Try to limit your daily intake of caffeine.

Stay hydrated. If you feel thirsty, your body is already getting dehydrated, so drink water often. Rehydrate your body with about eight cups of water a day, or more if you do a vigorous yoga practice that gets you sweaty. And don't overlook the importance of eating foods with water. Water-rich fruits and vegetables, for example, contribute to your daily hydration needs.

Eat lots of fruits, vegetables, and legumes. In addition to boosting your water intake, fruits and vegetables help fight chronic disease, in part because they're good sources of fiber, as are legumes. Plus, fruits and vegetables make great snacks, being much lower in calories than typical snack foods like chips and, most importantly, being much higher in nutrients.

Eat the right kinds of carbs. Some people have gotten swept up in a recent diet fad and have mostly sworn off eating carbs, but not all carbs are created equal. The right kinds of complex carbohydrates—such as whole grains and whole-grain products like bread or pasta—are good for the body. As they're digested they break down slowly, so they provide longer-lasting, more stable energy compared to sugar and refined carbohydrates.

THE PRACTICE OF WELLNESS

In the world of yoga, a healthy body and a healthy mind go hand in hand to create spiritual fulfillment. The physical practice of yoga offers great healing potential and health benefits. Yoga postures involve a lot of stretching, for example, which increases your overall flexibility and reduces muscular tension. Opening your body in this way also cultivates heat in the body, which aids in detoxification and expands your breath. The more deeply and easily, you're able to breathe, the more you increase vitality in your body by bringing oxygen to your muscles. You've probably noticed how exercise—whether it's a workout at the gym, brisk walking, or yoga—makes you feel more energetic.

It's important to spend a good amount of time in regular physical practice, not only for the outward benefits but also to strengthen your internal confidence, which may weaken if you have a negative relationship with your body. A solid practice also helps ward off harmful influences, such as the stresses of our technological world or toxins from food or the environment, all of which can lead to an unhealthy body—and mind and spirit.

In this chapter, you'll experience *kriyas* (purification practices) and *asanas* (yoga poses) in preparation for moving deeper toward your subtler areas of consciousness and awareness. Plan on incorporating the purification practices and yoga postures into your daily life as much as possible. It really isn't good enough to learn the routines here and then follow them only every now and then. Your goal should be to do the physical practices in this chapter three to four times per week, and preferably every day. That said, I know sometimes life gets in the way and daily practice isn't realistic, so just do what you can.

PURIFICATION PRACTICES

Purification practices, or kriyas, help clear and focus the mind while cleansing the physical body. The kriyas presented in this chapter allow you to fully benefit from the asanas, and also help reduce the potential for injury. For example, one purification practice is meant to cleanse your nasal passages. This is important because if your nasal cavities aren't clear, your yogic breathing will be hindered. The kriyas below fall into three categories:

1. Physical Purification
    - Candle Gaze to cleanse the eyes
    - Nasal Cleanse to clear the nasal passages

2. Breathing Purification
    - Uplifting Breath
    - Calming Breath

3. Relaxation Purification
    - Guided Body Scan and Relaxation

Whenever possible, please do all of the purification exercises before beginning any of the three posture sequences (beginner, intermediate, advanced) in this chapter. The entire purification regimen takes about 30 minutes to complete. If you're tight on time, do only the breathing and relaxation purifications, for at least half as long as the suggested time.

Take a brief rest between the kriyas and the asanas to fully calm your nervous system. Once your breathing is calm and you feel a sense of alert restfulness, you may begin your posture practice.

I'll offer just one caveat in regard to purification: Guard against staunch rituals around the purification of your body. Doing so may lead to tension, irritability, self-judgment, and just plain misery. Your main objective with regard to your physicality is to treat your body well; in addition to warding off disease, that also means living with zest and inspiration.

Avoid eating a large meal before practicing kriyas or asanas. Digesting food takes energy, and during your practice your body needs to focus its energy on the task at hand. Also, a full belly creates a sense of heaviness, which may restrict deep breathing and interfere with yoga movements such as twisting poses.

Physical Purification

— Candle Gaze (5 minutes) —

The purpose of this exercise is to calm the nervous system, cleanse the eyes, encourage concentration, and still the mind. It involves fixing your gaze on one point, such as a candle's flame. If you can't use a candle, a black dot on a white piece of paper will also work. And check your calendar: fixing your gaze on the full moon also works.

1. Sit in a comfortable cross-legged position on the floor or on a chair with your spine upright and long. If you sit cross-legged, ensure that your knees are lower than the top of your hip bones. If necessary, sit on a cushion or yoga bolster to achieve this position.

2. Ideally, you should have the candle's flame or the object of your attention at or slightly below eye-level. Sit across from the object, about 3 feet away.

3. Gaze at the flame for as long as you can without blinking, but avoid straining your eyes or squinting.

4. Maintain your focused attention on the flame for about 5 minutes and resist looking away.

— Nasal Cleanse (3 minutes) —

The nasal passages sometimes need to be cleansed beyond what's accomplished through normal breathing and nose blowing. This is where nasal cleansing using lightly salted water (also known as *jala neti*) can be beneficial. It keeps your breathing as clear as possible and also moistens the mucous membranes. However, if your nasal cavities are already blocked due to a cold, refrain from doing this purification practice until your nose is clear enough to breath normally.

During nasal cleansing, avoid sniffing or snorting the water; rather, allow it to gently flow through one nostril and out the other. It might feel strange to have water in your nose at first, but if you remain relaxed the sensation will begin to feel more comfortable. This practice is worth exploring because of its many benefits, which include helping curb allergies and sinus problems. The water's cooling effect also aids in alleviating headaches and migraines and discomfort associated with mental tension and depression. To perform nasal cleansing, you'll need the following supplies:

- A jala neti pot, available online or at new age, yoga, and natural food stores

- Sea salt

- Lukewarm water (at body temperature), purified if possible

I've provided instructions below, but if you're at all unsure about the technique, consult the instructions that came with your jala neti pot or search the Web, where you'll find instructional videos.

1. Nasal cleansing should be done over a sink or large bowl or in the yard. You can also do it in the shower.

2. Fill the jala neti pot with lukewarm saltwater, using one teaspoon of sea salt for every half liter of water (about two cups plus two tablespoons). The ratio is important, as it approximates the salinity of human blood. Mix thoroughly and ensure the salt is dissolved before use.

3. Insert the pot's spout into your right nostril, pointing the spout straight up so it's not blocked by the inside of your nose. The spout should fit tightly, forming a seal. Open your mouth and breathe gently through your mouth as you proceed. Don't breathe through your nose or swallow once the water starts flowing through your nasal passages.

4. Bend your body forward until the end of your nose is pointing toward the ground and tilt your head to the left so your left nostril is closer to the ground than any other part of your nose. Breathe through your mouth and allow about half of the pot of water to flow out through your left nostril.

5. Before switching sides, gently blow out through both nostrils to clear water and mucus from your nose, but don't blow hard, as you don't want to force water up into your sinuses or toward your ears. Wait 30 seconds, then repeat the process on the other side.

6. Repeat the cleansing sequence two times in each nostril, alternating nostrils each time.
◆

BREATHING PURIFICATION

Breathwork helps regulate energy levels in your body before you begin your practice of asanas. The two breathing purification exercises described below serve different purposes. The Uplifting Breath routine energizes your nervous system and boosts your body's overall energy level. The Calming Breath routine calms you and makes you feel rooted. People who feel depressed or have low energy will find the uplifting routine especially beneficial, and those who feel frenzied will find the grounding routine especially helpful. But please do both routines as part of your practice in the order that they're presented below. This will allow you to achieve optimally balanced energy.

— UPLIFTING BREATH (4 MINUTES) —

This breathing technique purifies the nasal passages and lungs, which helps the body eliminate excessive amounts of carbon dioxide and other impurities. It also improves digestion and activates and invigorates the spleen, pancreas, and abdominal muscles.

Avoid breathing through your mouth, as this can cause hyperventilation. Yoga breathing is done entirely through the nose. Also, please stop this purification exercise if you feel any kind of strain, and avoid it altogether if you have poor lung capacity, high blood pressure, or any discomfort, injury, or infection of the eyes or ears.

1. Sit in a comfortable cross-legged position on the floor or on a chair with your spine upright and long; avoid slouching. (If you sit cross-legged, remember to ensure that your knees are below the top of your hip bones. If necessary, sit on a cushion or yoga bolster to achieve this position.)

2. Begin exhaling slowly and deeply.

3. Inhale slowly, relaxing your abdomen. Allow your belly button to move away from your spine, so your belly is soft.

4. Exhale vigorously with a quick, strong blast of air. Contract your abdominal muscles by drawing your belly in. This will cause your diaphragm to rise, forcing air out of your lungs.

5. Pause for a split second after you breathe out, inhaling slightly during the pause. Repeat 4 to 8 short blasts of air on the exhale (you will be subtly inhaling between each blast). This completes 1 cycle.

6. Relax and take a few slow, natural breaths before beginning another cycle, remembering to breathe only through your nose at all times.

7. Each cycle lasts about 1 minute. If you're new to this routine, do 3 to 5 cycles, increasing the number you complete to a maximum of 7 cycles per day. It isn't a good idea to do more, as you could overstimulate your nervous system. ◆

— CALMING BREATH (8 MINUTES) —

This breathing practice cleanses the nervous system, strengthens the heart, clears the nostrils, lessens mental tension and worry, and helps alleviate headaches.

This practice requires open nasal cavities. Avoid doing it if your nose is congested from allergies or a cold. You don't want to gasp for air or inhale more oxygen through one nostril than the other.

Since this practice is done with your eyes closed, read through the procedure a few times to familiarize yourself with the process before you begin.

1. Sit cross-legged on the floor or on a chair with your spine upright and long. (If you sit cross-legged, remember to ensure that your knees are below the top of your hip bones. If necessary, sit on a cushion or yoga bolster to achieve this position.)

2. Be calm and close your eyes.

3. Close your right nostril with your right thumb. Inhale slowly through your left nostril, filling your lungs with air.

4. After a complete inhalation, close your left nostril with your ring finger on your right hand. Simultaneously open your right nostril.

5. Exhale slowly through your right nostril. After a complete exhalation, inhale through your right nostril, filling your lungs with air.

6. Close your right nostril by pressing it with your right thumb. Exhale through your left nostril, breathing out slowly. This completes 1 cycle. Think of each cycle as a horseshoe pattern: inhale on the left and exhale on the right, then inhale on the right and exhale on the left.

7. Complete 12 cycles. There is no restriction on how many cycles you do, because you can't overcalm your nervous system. The worst-case scenario is that you'll lull yourself to sleep! ◆

RELAXATION PURIFICATION

Making time for relaxation is vitally important for people living in the twenty-first century. Everything moves so fast these days! When everyone's in a rush, you're more likely to experience negative external influences during your day-to-day routine: cars honking, smog billowing, cell phones ringing, nonstop instant messaging, and the list goes on. You may feel as if you rarely if ever get a moment to just sit in peace. That's why I encourage you to relish the following guided body scan and make it part of your daily routine. This purification step is highly effective for bringing you calmness, quietness, and clarity.

— GUIDED BODY SCAN AND RELAXATION (10 MINUTES) —

This guided relaxation involves drawing awareness to different parts of your body without doing anything (such as moving your body or tensing and relaxing your muscles, as in progressive muscle relaxation). Simply use mental concentration to soften and relax any areas that feel tense. Wherever you find tension, visualize your breath moving into the area. The ultimate aim of this exercise is, above all, to create awareness of any tension you may have; your awareness is usually sufficient to allow you to let go of the tension.

Read the routine below a few times so you don't have to refer back to the guided script once you're lying down with your eyes closed. You can also go to my website (www.wadeimremorissette.com) and download a free MP3 audio file in which I gently talk you through the process. You can play the MP3 right off your computer or use a portable MP3 player.

For optimum results, create space and silence in your external environment and eliminate distractions as much as possible. To do the body scan, lie comfortably on your back. If lying on your back feels uncomfortable, sit in a chair. Begin by grounding yourself, then move on to the full body scan. As you proceed through the scan, focus on each body part for about one second.

GROUNDING METHOD —

1. Take a few deep breaths, exhaling fully and slowly each time.

2. Bring awareness to the surface of the skin on your body. Begin with your feet and move all the way up your torso, down your arms, and out your fingertips. Continue up your neck to the crown of your head.

3. Draw your attention back to your belly and navel. Take 12 breaths while focusing on your navel. Inhale, allowing your belly to rise. Exhale, allowing your belly to fall naturally.

4. Let your body become heavy, as if sinking into the floor. Surrender to the pull of gravity wherever you feel your body touching the floor. Soften your muscles and your bones, allowing your body to completely relax. Now you're ready to begin the guided body scan.

BODY SCAN METHOD —

1. Notice your feet. Notice your right foot. Become aware of your right heel, the arch of your right foot and the base of your toes. Notice the tip of your big toe, second toe, third toe, fourth toe, and little toe. Notice the top of your right foot, then notice your entire right foot and your right ankle.

2. Notice your left foot. Become aware of your left heel, the arch of your left foot, and the base of your toes. Notice the tip of your big toe, second toe, third toe, fourth toe, and little toe. Notice the top of your left foot, then notice your entire left foot and your left ankle.

3. Notice your right shin. Notice your right calf. Notice your right knee. Notice the back of your right knee. Notice your right thigh. Notice the back of your right thigh. Notice your right hip. Notice your right inner thigh.

4. Notice your left shin. Notice your left calf. Notice your left knee. Notice the back of your left knee. Notice your left thigh. Notice the back of your left thigh. Notice your left hip. Notice your left inner thigh.

5. Take your awareness to your pelvis. Then notice your navel. Notice your lower back. Notice your middle back. Notice your shoulder blades. Notice your upper back. Notice your solar plexus. Notice your chest.

6. Notice your right shoulder. Notice your right biceps and triceps. Notice your right elbow. Notice your right forearm. Notice your right wrist. Notice the palm of your right hand. Notice your right thumb, your index finger, your middle finger, your ring finger, and your pinky. Notice the top of your right hand. Notice your entire right hand, front and back.

7. Notice your left shoulder. Notice your left biceps and triceps. Notice your left elbow. Notice your left forearm. Notice your left wrist. Notice the palm of your left hand. Notice your left thumb, your index finger, your middle finger, your ring finger, and your pinky. Notice the top of your left hand. Notice your entire left hand, front and back.

8. Notice your throat. Notice the front and back of your throat. Notice the sides of your neck. Notice the back of your neck. Notice your skull, scalp, and head. Notice the crown of your head. Notice your forehead. Notice your eyebrows. Notice your eyelashes. Notice your eye sockets. Notice your eyeballs. Notice your nose. Notice your right nostril. Notice your left nostril. Notice your lips. Notice your chin. Notice your jaw.

9. Notice your entire face. Notice your right ear. Notice your left ear.

10. Notice your neck to the crown of your head. Notice your torso. Notice your right arm and hand. Notice your left arm and hand. Notice your belly.

11. As you inhale, let your belly rise slightly without strain. As you exhale let your belly fall.

12. Lie quietly for 3 minutes.

13. Slowly get up. Drink a glass of water before moving to your asana practice. ◆

POSTURE PRACTICE

This section focuses on yoga poses, also called postures or asanas. The routines on the following pages were designed to bring your focus inward as you strengthen and limber up your muscles. Practicing asanas offers many benefits. Here are just a few of them:

- Keeping your body strong and supple as you age

- Increasing your energy and vitality

- Releasing toxins and tensions from your body

- Strengthening your internal systems against disease

■ Helping you maintain a healthy weight

Yoga also has the ability to slow you down mentally, even when the world around you feels like it's moving at a breakneck pace. So as you perform the sequences that follow, think of your practice as a way to help you cope with the external stressors of modern living.

DOING THE POSTURES

I've included three sequences: one for beginners, one for intermediate practitioners, and one for advanced yogis. Perform the sequence appropriate for you once or twice daily up to six days per week. Each routine takes about 30 to 45 minutes to complete. If you don't have that much time, consider working in a shorter routine when you can, versus doing long but only occasional sessions. To make a routine shorter, perform it from start to finish only one or two times instead of the suggested three or four times.

Practicing for ten minutes every day is more beneficial than practicing once a week for ninety minutes because when you aren't practicing, you move farther away from your inner sensibilities. A short daily practice does more to recharge your batteries or keep you connected to your subtle energies than longer sessions with long breaks in between.

If you're relatively new to yoga or haven't practiced it in a while, start with the beginner sequence. If you have a moderate amount of experience doing yoga, you may wish to try the intermediate sequence first, then work your way up to the advanced program. When a posture feels too challenging for you to complete, do what you can, then move on to the next pose. It's not necessary to master all the postures in this book right away—after all, yoga is a lifelong journey.

In any of the three sequences, perform the poses and the transitions between poses slowly and with patience. The instructions indicate how long to hold each pose, generally in terms of a number of breaths. One breath equals one inhalation and one exhalation. The number of breaths you take in each pose will depend on your experience level and what you'd like to get out of the practice. For example, the longer you hold a pose, the longer your overall workout and the more you work on muscular strength. The less time you hold a pose, the quicker the workout and the more you experience a continuous flow of movement, which increases the cardiovascular intensity of your practice. However, to reap the health benefits of true cardiovascular exercise, complement your yoga practice with aerobic activities such as brisk walking, jogging, cycling, and swimming.

YOGA BREATHING

Yoga postures must always be accompanied with breath through the nose, not the mouth. Without coordinated yoga breath, called *ujjayi*, you're simply stretching. Yoga breathing is diaphragmatic; think of breathing down into your lower belly. Ujjayi breath sounds like the ocean flowing in and out, or the way Darth Vader from Star Wars sounds when he breathes. This type of breathing is meant to uplift you.

The instructions often indicate when to inhale and exhale. Whenever this isn't indicated, simply breathe slowly and naturally. Always breathe before you begin movement and continue yogic breathing during the pose. In other words, whenever you're moving, you should also be breathing. The diagram below helps illustrate this process; as you can see, movement is always encompassed within the flow of the breath. For the Relaxation Pose, there's no movement and the goal of the pose is relaxation, so simply breathe naturally.

_____ Breath

_____ Movement

EQUIPMENT YOU NEED

Yoga doesn't require much in the way of expensive equipment. For the postures presented in this book, please have the following items. All of them are available online or in yoga stores, or in many book stores and fitness apparel shops:

- **A yoga mat.** If you sweat during yoga, select one that provides good traction for your feet. You can also lay a towel on top of your yoga mat if it becomes slippery with sweat.

- **A yoga bolster or block.** You can place either of these under your buttocks to allow you to sit in cross-legged or lotus positions more comfortably. They will make certain poses more comfortable if you aren't very flexible. For example, if your hand doesn't reach the floor in the Triangle pose, you can rest it on a yoga block until you become flexible enough to reach the floor.

- **Folded blankets or a cushion.** In many cases, you can use blankets or regular cushions as you would a yoga bolster or blocks.

- **A yoga or stretching strap.** You can use the strap to assist with stretching and alignment during shoulder stretches and seated forward bends.

- **Lightweight clothing that isn't restrictive.** You may also want a warm shirt or blanket for when you lie in relaxation at the end of your practice.

Finding a Local Yoga Teacher

In addition to following the sequences in this book, I encourage you to find a local yoga teacher to ensure your interpretations of the poses on these pages are correct. A live teacher can help you make adjustments that will greatly enhance and evolve your personal practice; sometimes even very minor changes make a big difference. You'll notice that each teacher has her or her own style, angle, or theme when it comes to properly practicing the postures. Try a variety of teachers and classes to decide what method and instructional style resonates most with you.

POSTURE SEQUENCES AND DESCRIPTIONS

On the following pages you'll find a warm-up routine, two versions of the sun salutation, and then three sequences of asanas: beginner, intermediate, and advanced, each with a core phase and then a sequence for cooldown and integration. While you're learning the poses in each sequence, please read the step-by-step instructions on how to do each pose before attempting the posture. After each description, I offer one or more tips to help you refine the posture. This will help you direct your awareness to the right areas or make adjustments that will lead to a more effective practice. I also include directions for modifying some of the poses so they feel easier or accommodate various abilities. If a posture feels too challenging or uncomfortable, please modify it or skip it. Once you're familiar with all of the poses in a sequence, transition smoothly from each pose to the next, in one long, continuous flow.

In each pose, feel for what's often called "the edge"—the point where you begin to feel a stronger sensation in the pose (perhaps a deeper stretch) and your breath begins to change. Experiencing the physical sensation of the edge will help you experience maximum benefits while avoiding injury. Explore the edge in each posture because this is the point where your body begins to open and flexibility increases, but to avoid injury be mindful not to go beyond the edge. Be curious about it, but don't push it.

There's a lot to learn in the rest of the chapter. As you're getting started, what's most important is to practice carefully and with intention. You may need to build your practice up in small steps. For example, the first day you might learn the purification practices. The next day you could learn the warm-up sequence. You might want to stick with just those two elements for several days, until they're familiar. Then keep those practices going as you move on to learning the sun salutation. Once you've got that down, start learning the poses in the beginner sequence. The sequence is designed for optimum flow and balance, but if it's too much to learn all at once, try a few asanas from the core phase and be sure to

Posture Classifications

There are various classifications of yoga postures, and some categories are more difficult than others. Each category has different purposes and produces different effects, as described below. Refer to the appendix for lists of how all of the postures in this book are categorized.

Seated: Grounding, meditative

Supine: Relaxing, restorative, calming to the nervous system

Forward bending: Calming, relieves back tension, alleviates anxiety or worry

Backward bending: Stretches the chest, shoulders, or back of the body, strengthens and aligns the spine, counteracts low vitality and depression, opens the chest, invigorates

Twisting: Promotes spinal health, relieves back tension, stretches the torso, upper back, shoulders, or neck

Balancing: Balances the right and left sides of the brain, activates the core

Standing: Invigorates, improves strength, stamina, and stability

Inverted: Restorative, rests the heart, alleviates headaches, flushes the internal organs follow up with a few from the cooldown and integration sequence. Within a week or two, you should be able to put the entire sequence together, from purification to cooldown.

WARM-UP —

A proper warm-up prepares you mentally for the workout ahead. It also lubricates your joints and warms up your muscles so there's less risk of injury.

1. Mountain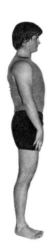

2. Child's Pose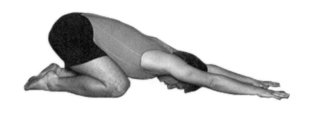

3. Cow and Cat

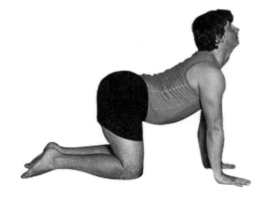 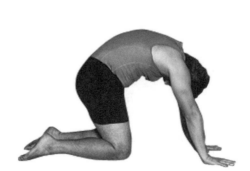

4. Downward Dog (to Gazing Halfway Up)

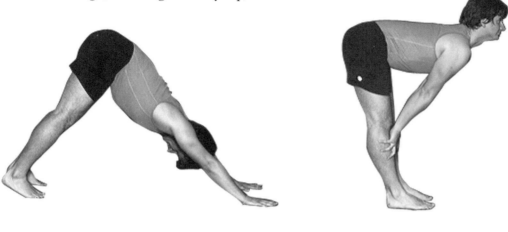

5. Standing Forward Bend
   (to Extended Mountain to Mountain) ◆

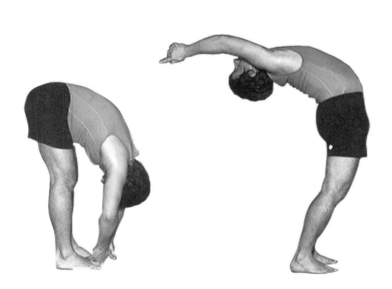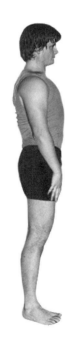

— 1. MOUNTAIN —

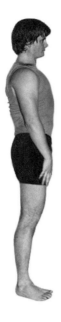

Mountain is one of yoga's base postures. You will return to this pose often during your practice because it's symmetrical—all parts are equal. While it might seem as if this pose requires you to just stand in place, you'll see from the description below and your own practice that it involves many physical subtleties. Because many poses begin or end in **Mountain**, when doing a sequence of yoga postures, **Mountain** is often a transition. You can move through this position without pausing; or, if you need to recenter yourself or rest a bit, you can remain in **Mountain** for several breaths.

1. Stand with your feet touching each other, hip-width apart, or somewhere between those two stances. Your feet should be parallel and your heels aligned. Evenly distribute your weight through the bottom of both feet, and don't lean forward or back.

2. Make sure your hips are over your knees and your knees are over your ankles, in one line of energy.

3. Lift up through your hips and tuck your tailbone under slightly.

4. Lift your chest slightly.

5. Rest your arms at your sides and roll your shoulders up toward your ears, and then back and down.

6. Tuck your chin slightly or hold it parallel to the floor. Lift through the back of your neck. Breathe and hold the position for 3 breaths. ◆

Tips: Align your ears over your shoulders, your shoulders over your hips, and your hips over your ankles. Women have structurally wider pelvises than men (for childbirth), so women's feet may be slightly wider apart during this pose.

— 2. Child's Pose —

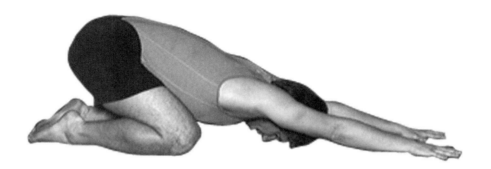

1. Get on your hands and knees, with your big toes touching.

2. As you exhale, bring your buttocks to your heels and allow your forehead to rest on the floor. Place your arms by your sides or stretch them over your head with your palms on the floor.

3. Breathe into the back of your body, from your lower back to your shoulder blades, and hold the position for 3 breaths.

4. To release, come back to all fours, with your knees aligned under your hips and your wrists aligned under your shoulders. ✦

Tips: Soften your back and allow your mental focus to be drawn inward. If you're heavy or have large breasts, you can place your knees wider apart, but do keep your big toes together. If your buttocks don't touch your heels, you can ease any potential knee strain by placing a bolster or yoga block under your buttocks if you like.

— 3. COW AND CAT —

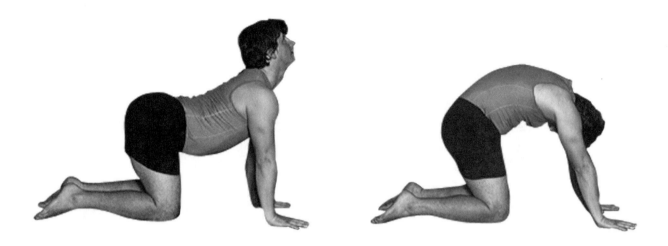

1. From the all-fours position, inhale and drop your belly toward the floor, arching your back. Lift your chest away from your belly button. Gaze ahead and slightly up. This is the **Cow** pose.

2. As you exhale, press your hands into the floor and draw your belly in as you round your back. Draw your chin toward your throat. This is the **Cat** pose.

3. Repeat for 5 to 7 cycles. ✦

Tips: In the **Cow** pose, focus on elongating your spine to avoid overarching your back. In the **Cat** pose, draw your belly button in toward your spine as far as possible and press firmly through your arms.

— 4. DOWNWARD DOG —

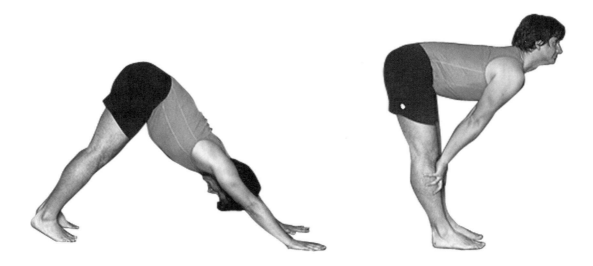

1. Still in the all-fours position, make sure your knees and feet are about hip-width apart.

2. Keeping your palms firmly on the floor, curl your toes under, then exhale and lift your sit bones toward the ceiling, straightening your legs.

3. Gaze through your extended legs and spread your fingers and toes wide. Press through the balls of your feet at the base of your big toes and through your thumbs and index fingers.

4. Hold for 3 to 5 breaths. Each time you inhale, expand your rib cage. Each time you exhale, pull your belly in.

5. To release, exhale and step your feet up to a position between your hands, with knees bent if necessary. Straighten your legs, keeping your hands on the floor or resting them on your ankles or shins. Gaze halfway up directly in front of you, elongating and gently arching your spine. Keep your neck long. (This transitional position is the pose **Gazing Halfway** Up.) ✦

Tips: Draw your sit bones as high as possible while pressing your heels toward the floor. Keep a neutral spine in **Downward Dog**, avoiding rounding or overarching your back. If you feel a lot of weight in your shoulders, bend your knees, draw your sit bones upward as high as you can, then slowly straighten your legs. Allow your heart region to sink slightly, then begin extending through your arms and sides.

— 5. STANDING FORWARD BEND —

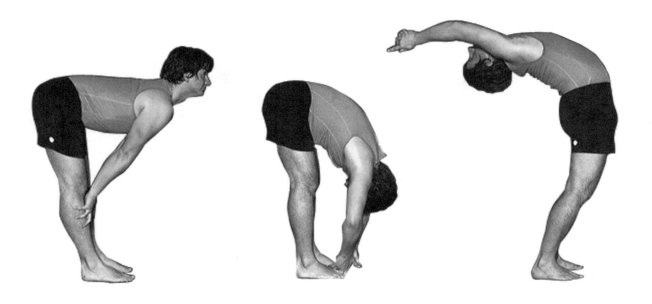

1. From **Gazing Halfway Up**, exhale, relax your neck and back, and bring your chest and belly button toward your legs.

2. Place your hands on your shins, ankles, or feet, or on the floor, as you are able. Soften the back of your neck. Hold for 3 to 5 breaths.

3. To release, inhale and hinge upward from your hips, reaching your arms to the sides, then overhead, as you return to standing. Extend back into a gentle arch, pressing your hips forward to keep them aligned over your ankles. (This transitional position is the pose **Extended Mountain**.) Then exhale and return to **Mountain**. ✦

Tips: In the forward bend, make sure your weight doesn't fall too far back on your heels. To correct for this, bend your legs, lean into the base of your toes, then straighten your legs.

SUN SALUTATIONS

After you do the warm-up sequence, do several sun salutations to further warm and energize your body. As you'll see from the images and descriptions on the following pages, sun salutations are a series of asanas. However, in sun salutations the poses are dynamically linked in one continuous flow, rather than each being held for several breaths. With one exception, the Soft Sun Salutation is comprised of poses in the warm-up sequence, which you've already learned. Since the movements are very basic, it isn't necessary to learn all of the subtleties of each pose in order to do sun salutations. But as you become more accomplished at the individual poses, you'll be able to bring more intention to your practice of sun salutations.

I've included two versions of the sun salutation: the Soft Sun Salutation and the Strength Sun Salutation. When you're first getting started with practicing yoga, do two or three Soft Sun Salutations. As you progress, begin to include the Strength Sun Salutation for one or two repetitions and increase the overall number of repetitions until, at the advanced level, you're doing five repetitions of the Strength Sun Salutation.

SOFT SUN SALUTATION SUMMARY —

1. Mountain

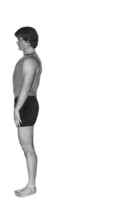

2. Extended Mountain

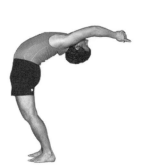

3. Standing Forward Bend

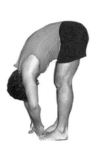

4. Gazing Halfway Up

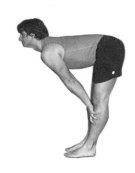

5. Flag (right leg back)

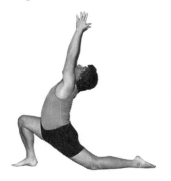

6. Downward Dog

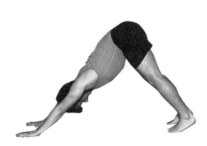

7. Flag (left leg back)

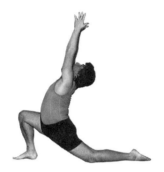

8. Gazing Halfway Up

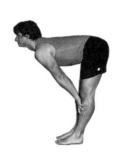

9. Standing Forward Bend

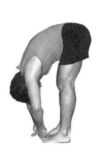

10. Extended Mountain

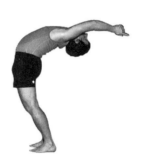

11. Mountain ◆

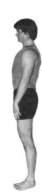

SOFT SUN SALUTATION —

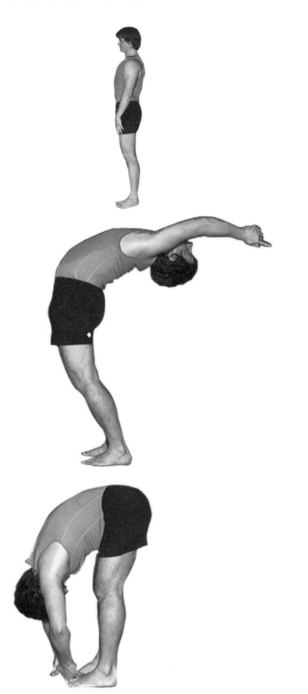

1. Begin in **Mountain.**

2. **Extended Mountain:** As you inhale, reach your arms up over your head, shoulder-distance apart, and extend back into a gentle arch.

3. **Standing Forward Bend:** As you exhale, hinge forward from your hips and place your hands on your shins, ankles, or feet, or on the floor, as you are able. Drop your head and soften the back of your neck.

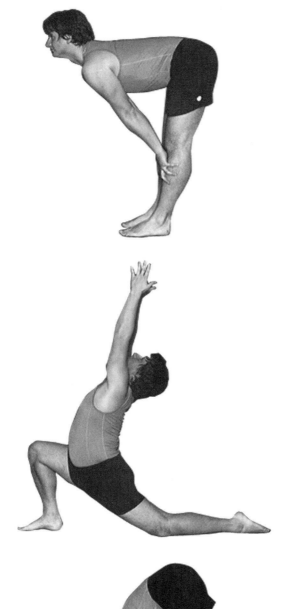

4. **Gazing Halfway Up:** Inhale and gaze halfway up directly in front of you, elongating your spine and working toward a slight arch if you're able.

5. **Flag (right leg back):** Exhale and step your right foot back into a lunge position, making sure your left knee is aligned over your ankle. Your feet should be about the same distance apart as the length of one of your legs, and your weight should be centered between your feet, not in your hands. Inhale and reach your arms overhead, palms facing each other. If this position is too difficult at first, place your hands on your hips and lift your chest toward the ceiling, keeping your shoulders back.

6. **Downward Dog:** Exhale and place your hands on the floor, shoulder-distance apart, one hand on either side of your front foot. Step your left foot back alongside your right foot, lifting your sit bones up toward the ceiling and gazing through your extended legs.

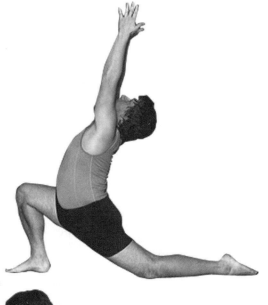

7. **Flag (left leg back):** Inhale and step your right foot forward into a lunge position, making sure your right knee is aligned over your ankle. With that same inhale, reach your arms overhead, palms facing each other; alternatively, place your hands on your hips and lift your chest toward the ceiling, keeping your shoulders back. If you need to, take an extra breath in this position before transitioning to **Gazing Halfway Up**.

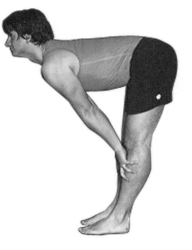

8. **Gazing Halfway Up:** Exhale, place your hands on either side of your right foot, shoulder-distance apart, and step your left foot forward, alongside your right foot. Straighten your legs, keeping your hands on the floor or placing them on your shins, ankles, or feet. Inhale and gaze halfway up directly in front of you, elongating your spine and working toward a slight arch.

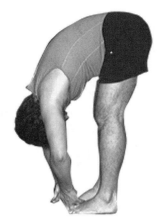

9. **Standing Forward Bend:** Exhale, relax your neck and back, and bring your chest and belly button toward your legs.

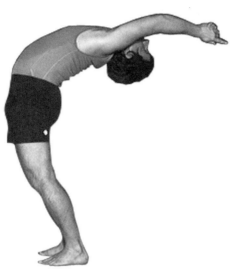

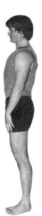

10. **Extended Mountain:** Inhale and return to an upright position, keeping your spine long and sweeping your arms up over your head, shoulder-distance apart. Extend back into a gentle arch.

11. **Mountain:** Exhale and return to Mountain, with your arms by your sides. ✦

STRENGTH SUN SALUTATION SUMMARY —

1. Mountain

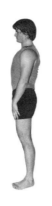

2. Extended Mountain

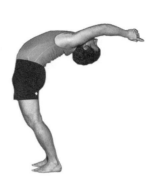

3. Standing Forward Bend

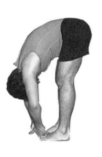

4. Gazing Halfway Up

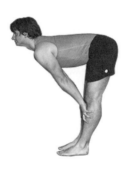

5. Long Staff

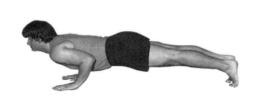

6. Upward Dog

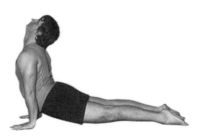

7. Downward Dog

8. Gazing Halfway Up

9. Standing Forward Bend

10. Extended Mountain

11. Mountain ◆

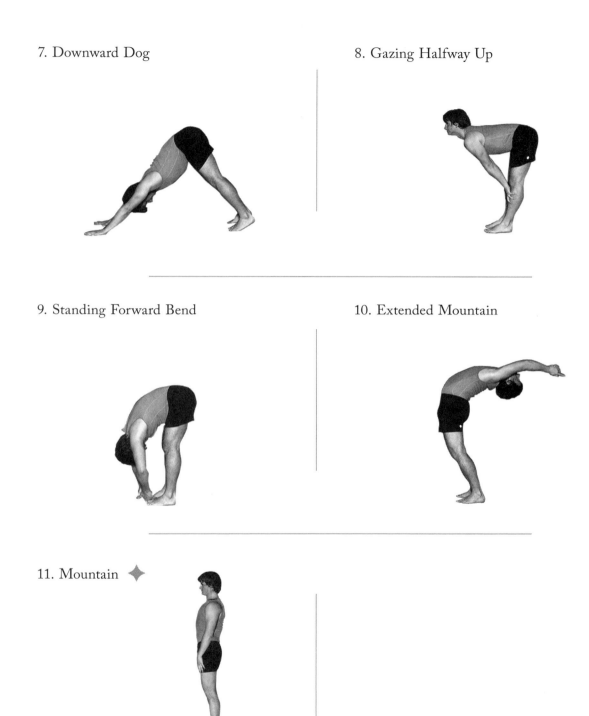

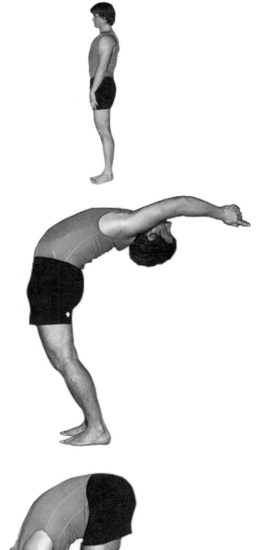

1. Begin in **Mountain**.

2. **Extended Mountain:** As you inhale, reach your arms up over your head, shoulder-distance apart, and extend back into a gentle arch.

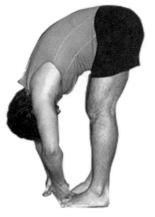

3. **Standing Forward Bend:** As you exhale, hinge forward from your hips and place your hands on your shins, ankles, or feet, or on the floor, as you are able. Drop your head and soften the back of your neck.

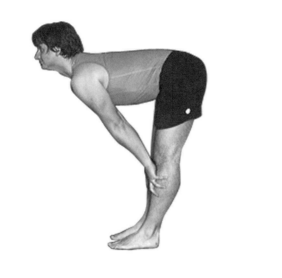

4. **Gazing Halfway Up:** Inhale and gaze halfway up directly in front of you, elongating your spine and working toward a slight arch if you're able.

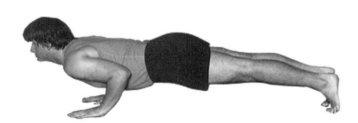

5. **Long Staff:** Exhale and, with your hands on the ground shoulder-width apart, step your feet back behind you, hip-distance apart, so that your body is in one straight line; think of it as a horizontal version of **Mountain**, with your knees, hips, and shoulders aligned. Bend your elbows, keeping them by your sides, to lower your body a few inches above the ground. Gaze forward and keep your thigh muscles engaged and your belly in.

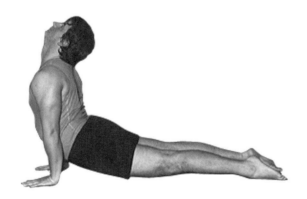

6. **Upward Dog:** As you inhale, lift and press your chest forward and up, dropping your shoulder blades to keep your shoulders back and down and keeping the tops of your toes and feet on the floor.

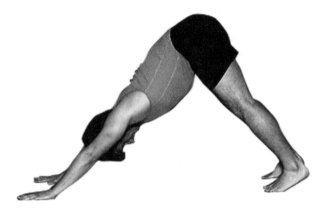

7. **Downward Dog:** Exhale, curl your toes under, and lift your sit bones up toward the ceiling, straightening your legs. Keep your back long and gaze through your extended legs.

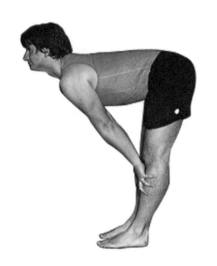

8. **Gazing Halfway Up:** Inhale and step your feet up to a position between your hands, with knees bent if necessary. Straighten your legs, keeping your hands on the floor or resting them on your ankles or shins. Gaze halfway up directly in front of you, elongating and gently arching your spine.

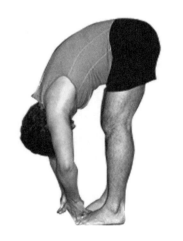

9. **Standing Forward Bend:** Exhale, relax your neck and back, and bring your chest and belly button toward your legs.

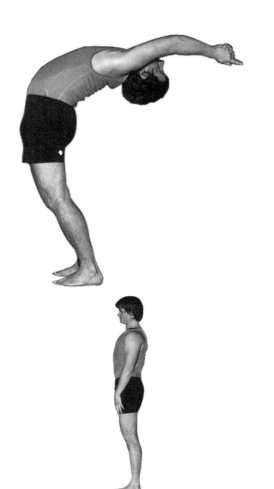

10. **Extended Mountain:** Inhale and return to an upright position, keeping your spine long and sweeping your arms up over your head, shoulder-distance apart. Extend back into a gentle arch.

11. **Mountain:** Exhale and return to Mountain, with your arms by your sides. ✦

BEGINNER PRACTICE OVERVIEW

Once you're familiar with the warm-up sequence and the Soft Sun Salutation, you can start working on the beginner sequence outlined below. Because the poses in the core sequence, cooldown, and integration balance and build upon one another, it's best to do the entire sequence. However, if you're new to yoga or need to build strength and flexibility, it's fine to learn a few new poses from the core phase and cooldown and integration, below, during each session until you've learned all of them. As soon as you're ready, you can put the entire beginner program together:

1. **Physical purification:** At a minimum, practice Uplifting Breath for 2 minutes and Calming Breath for 4 minutes, then do the Guided Body Scan and Relaxation for at least 5 minutes.

2. **Warm-up:** Do the complete warm-up sequence.

3. **Sun salutations:** Do up to three repetitions of Soft Sun Salutation.

4. **Beginner sequence:** Do the core phase and cooldown and integration outlined below. In the core phase, when you return to Mountain at the end of each pose, you can pause for a breath or two to center yourself or rest before proceeding. Once you become very familiar with the full descriptions, you can use the sequence summary as a quick reference.

BEGINNER SEQUENCE SUMMARY
BEGINNER CORE PHASE —

1. Triangle (to Mountain)

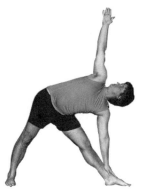

2. Warrior 2 (to Mountain)

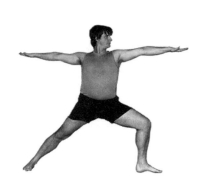

3. Wide-Leg Forward Bend (to Mountain)

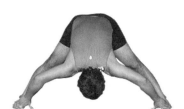

4. Exalted Warrior (to Mountain)

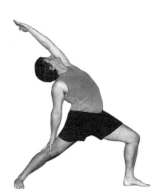

5. Tree (to Mountain) ✦

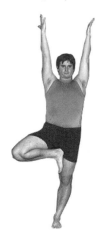

BEGINNER COOLDOWN AND INTEGRATION —

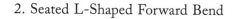

1. Beginner Accomplished Pose

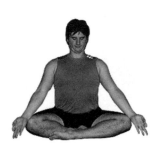

2. Seated L-Shaped Forward Bend

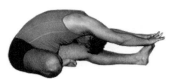

3. Seated Twist

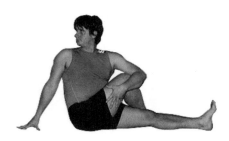

4. Seated L-Shaped Side Bend

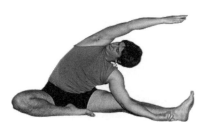

5. Table

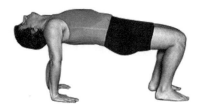

6. Supine Flexion

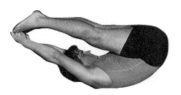

7. Bridge

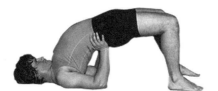

8. Both-Legs-Up Recline

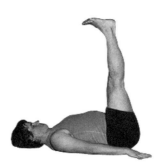

9. Knee-Down Twist

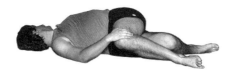

10. Knees to Chest

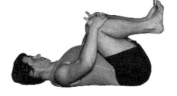

11. Relaxation Pose ◆

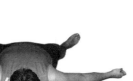

— 1. TRIANGLE —

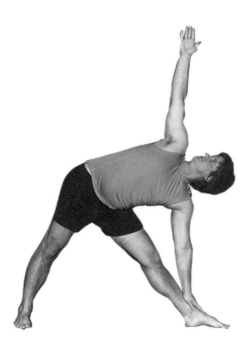

1. Begin in **Mountain**.

2. Inhale and step your right foot back. Your feet should be about the same distance apart as the length of one of your legs.

3. Exhale and rotate your body 90 degrees to the right, keeping your left foot facing directly left and turning your right foot so that it's pointing slightly left, rather than directly toward the long side of the mat.

4. Inhale and extend your arms to the sides with your hands slightly higher than your shoulders.

5. Exhale and bend sideways to the left, keeping your spine long, until your left hand touches your shin, ankle, or toes. With your right arm and hand pointing directly toward the ceiling, rotate your rib cage and chest up toward the ceiling, keeping your spine long. Hold for 5 to 12 breaths.

6. To release, inhale, contract the muscles in your right thigh, and activate your core as you bring your torso upright, arms once again out to the sides.

7. Remaining in this stance, rotate your left foot to point slightly inward, toward your right heel and point your right foot directly to the right (to the back of the mat), then repeat steps 5 and 6 on the opposite side.

8. Rotate 90 degrees to the left, with your feet and hips facing the front of the mat, then step your right leg forward into **Mountain**. ◆

Tips: Keep your shoulders soft by dropping the tops of your shoulders down from the ears.

— 2. WARRIOR 2 —

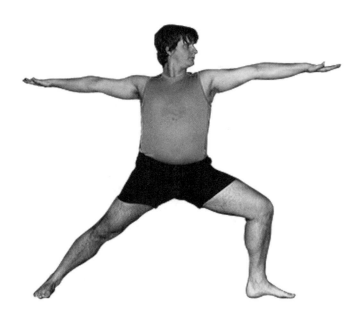

1. From **Mountain,** inhale and step your right foot back. Your feet should be about the same distance apart as the length of one of your legs.

2. Exhale and rotate your body 90 degrees to the right, keeping your left foot facing directly left and turning your right foot so that it's pointing slightly left, rather than directly toward the long side of the mat.

3. Inhale and extend your arms to the sides at shoulder height.

4. Exhale and bend your left leg, aligning your left knee over your left ankle. Your leg should be bent to about 90 degrees.

5. Gaze at your left arm, keeping your torso centered over your legs and your arms extended equally on either side. Lift your chest and drop your shoulders away from your ears. Lower your shoulder blades toward your hips. Hold for 5 to 12 breaths.

6. To release, inhale, contract the muscles in your right thigh, and activate your core as you straighten your left leg and gaze straight ahead.

7. Rotate your left foot to point slightly inward, toward your right heel, and point your right foot directly to the right (to the back of the mat), then repeat steps 4 through 6 on the opposite side.

8. Rotate 90 degrees to the left, with your feet and hips facing the front of the mat, then step your right leg forward into **Mountain**. ✦

Tips: Look down at the leg that's bent; you should be able to see your knee aligned between your big toe and second toe.

— 3. Wide-Leg Forward Bend —

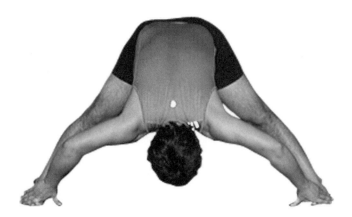

1. From **Mountain**, inhale and step your right foot back. Your feet should be about the same distance apart as the length of one of your legs.

2. Exhale and rotate your body 90 degrees to the right, with your toes pointing toward the long side of your mat or turned slightly inward.

3. Inhale and raise your arms overhead, palms facing each other.

4. Exhale and hinge forward from your hips. Place your hands on your feet or on the floor so they're aligned under your shoulders.

5. Lengthen your spine, allowing the crown of your head to drop toward the floor, and gaze between your legs. Hold for 5 to 12 breaths.

6. To release, inhale and look halfway up as you bring your hands to your hips. Exhale. Inhale again and reach your arms all the way up as you hinge back up from your hips to return to standing.

7. Exhale and bring your hands back down to your sides as you rotate 90 degrees to the left, with your feet and hips facing the front of the mat, then step your right leg forward into **Mountain**. ✦

Tips: For a more challenging option, bring your hands together behind your back and interlace your fingers, then try to straighten your arms and extend them toward the ceiling, working toward bringing them over and beyond your head.

— 4. Exalted Warrior —

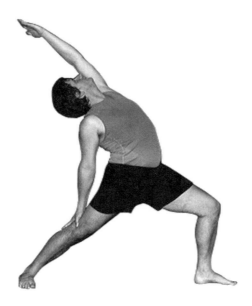

1. From **Mountain**, inhale and step your right leg back. Your feet should be about the same distance apart as the length of one of your legs, with your right leg turned slightly out. Draw your left hip back and push your right hip forward to maintain good alignment.

2. Exhale and bend your left leg, aligning the knee over your left ankle. Your leg should be bent to about 90 degrees.

3. Inhale and slide your right hand down your right leg, avoiding putting extra weight onto the leg with your hand. Then reach your left arm up and back as you rotate your chest up toward the ceiling. Hold for 5 to 12 breaths.

4. To release, inhale, contract the muscles in your right thigh, and activate your core as you straighten your left leg and return to an upright position, gazing straight ahead.

5. Rotate 180 degrees to the right, with your hips and right foot facing the right (the back of the mat) and your left foot turned slightly out. Repeat steps 2 through 4 on the opposite side.

6. Rotate 180 degrees to the left, with your hips and feet facing the front of the mat, and step your right leg forward into **Mountain**. ✦

Tips: Elongate and stretch into the extension of your spine.

— 5. TREE —

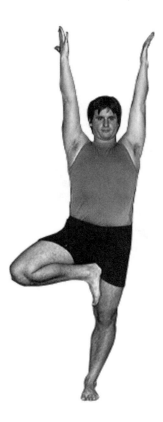

1. From **Mountain**, shift your weight onto your left leg. Bend your right leg, lifting your foot off the floor, and place the sole of your right foot on the inside of your left calf or left thigh (not the knee).

2. As you inhale, bring your hands to chest height and place your palms together. You may also reach your arms overhead, palms facing one another.

3. Keep your hips and shoulders facing forward by drawing your left hip back and pushing your right hip forward. Work on staying balanced as you hold for 5 to 12 breaths.

4. To release, exhale and bring your bent leg toward your chest, knee up, then inhale and lower the leg to the floor. If you need to, rest and recenter in **Mountain** for 1 breath.

5. Repeat on the opposite side. ◆

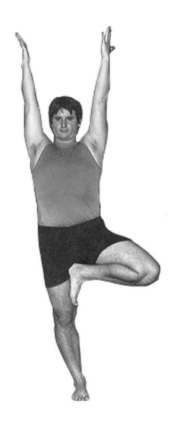

Tips: Keep your chin slightly tucked in and lengthen through your rib cage. To help maintain your balance, keep your awareness on your belly button and the midline of your body.

— 1. BEGINNER ACCOMPLISHED POSE —

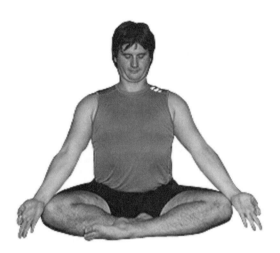

1. Sit cross-legged on the floor.

2. Bring your right heel slightly to the left of the midline of your body and your left heel slightly to the right of the midline of your body. Press your thighs toward the floor.

3. Hold your spine upright and long and either keep your chin parallel to the floor or tuck it slightly. Hold for 5 to 12 breaths. ◆

Tips: Pressing your thighs toward the floor may be hard at first, as it opens your pelvis and requires flexibility. With repeated practice, it will get easier. If your knees are higher than the top of your hip bones, sit on a bolster or cushion to allow your pelvis to rotate forward.

— 2. Seated L-Shaped Forward Bend —

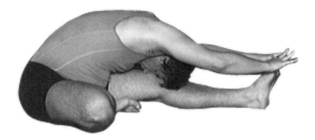

1. Still seated on the floor, extend your legs in front of you and use your hands to pull the flesh of your buttocks toward the back of the mat; this will help ground your sit bones on the mat and allow a forward rotation of your pelvis.

2. Bend your right leg, working your right heel toward your groin. Your left leg should be aligned straight out from your left hip.

3. As you inhale, reach your arms overhead.

4. Exhale and lean forward, drawing your belly button toward your thigh and working your chin toward your shin and the crown of your head toward your toes. Hold for 5 to 12 breaths.

5. To release, inhale and bring your arms overhead as you lift your chest and extend your right leg, then exhale and rest your arms beside your body.

6. Repeat on the opposite side. ◆

Tips: Keep your sit bones on the ground and your chest lifted as you hinge forward. Keep the thigh on the straight leg aligned by rotating it toward your body's midline. If you need a slightly easier variation until you're more flexible, slightly bend the extended leg.

— 3. SEATED TWIST —

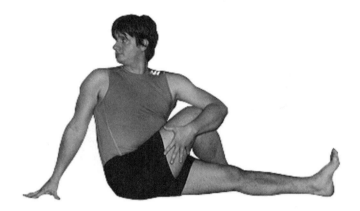

1. Still sitting with your legs extended, bend your right leg, placing your right heel to the left side of your left outer thigh, with the base of your toes firmly rooted on the floor.

2. Inhale and lift your left arm up overhead.

3. Exhale and hug your right knee with your left elbow, reaching your right hand behind you and placing it on the floor close to your tailbone.

4. Inhale and rotate to the right, lengthening the left side of your body and your spine.

5. Exhale and press your left elbow against the outside of your right leg, using your elbow as a lever to deepen the posture. Hold for 5 to 12 breaths.

6. To release, inhale and gaze back to the center, bringing yourself out of the twist, then extend your right leg alongside your left leg.

7. Repeat on the opposite side. ◆

Tips: The spine loves to twist when there's space between the vertebrae. Stay long in your spine and think of twisting from your middle back, as the lumbar spine has very little mobility for this kind of motion.

— 4. SEATED L-SHAPED SIDE BEND —

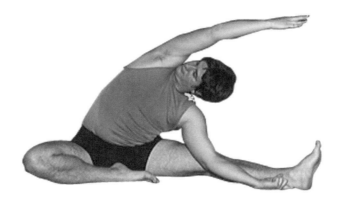

1. Still sitting with your legs extended, bend your right leg, working your right heel toward your groin and placing the outside of your right thigh and calf on the floor. Then take your left leg 30 degrees to the left.

2. As you exhale, bend to the left and place your left elbow on the floor just inside your left leg, keeping your spine elongated.

3. Inhale and rotate your torso and chest toward the ceiling as you extend your right arm up over your head and toward your left foot. Hold for 5 to 12 breaths.

4. To release, inhale, extend both legs forward, and return to an upright, forward-facing position with your shoulders square to the front of the mat and your arms by your sides.

5. Repeat on the opposite side. ✦

Tips: Rotate through your chest and rib cage on the side you're stretching toward the ceiling. If it's difficult for you to reach your elbow to the floor, bend your straight leg as much as needed to allow the elbow to comfortably touch the floor.

— 5. TABLE —

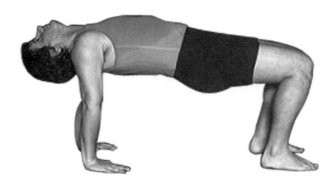

1. Still sitting with your legs extended, ensure that your ankles and big toes are touching or just slightly apart.

2. Place your hands on the floor on either side of your hips, fingers pointing toward your feet and wrists aligned under your shoulders.

3. As you inhale, contract your thigh muscles and lift your pelvis off the floor, balancing on your hands and feet. The alignment of your body should be similar to a horizontal version of **Mountain**, with your knees, hips, and shoulders aligned. Try not to let your hips fall from that line. Hold for 5 to 12 breaths.

4. Each time you exhale, press your feet into the floor, draw your belly in while keeping your pelvis lifted, and tuck your chin into your chest. Each time you inhale, think of lifting your pelvis to maintain good alignment.

5. To release, lower your buttocks to the floor between your hands, tucking your chin into your chest at the same time. ◆

Tips: Once you've practiced this pose for a while and have greater strength, allow the front of your neck to completely lengthen so that you're looking slightly back.

— 6. Supine Flexion —

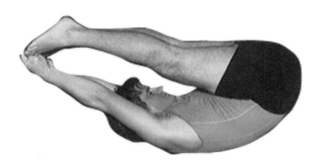

1. Lie on your back with your arms by your sides.

2. As you exhale, bring your extended legs up to 90 degrees, pressing into your palms to help with the lifting motion, then lift your tailbone and continue rolling up through your spine until the weight of your body is on your upper back and shoulders, but not your neck. Your head should be resting on the floor with your neck relaxed.

3. With your legs bent or straight, wrap your hands around your lower legs or ankles, or gently grasp your toes. Hold for 5 to 12 breaths.

4. To release, roll down through your spine until your lower back and tailbone are on the floor, drawing your belly in to keep your abs tight. Bend both knees, then lower one leg at a time back down to the floor and lie with your legs extended and arms by your sides.

Tips: While in the pose, work on straightening your legs and lengthening your upper spine against the mat.

— 7. BRIDGE —

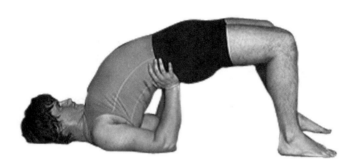

1. Still lying on your back with your palms on the floor, bend your legs so your ankles are under your knees, toes pointing straight ahead.

2. As you inhale, press your palms into the floor and lift your tailbone up off the floor, then continue curling through your spine until your middle back and upper back are up off the floor.

3. Keep your palms on the floor, interlace your fingers and extend your arms underneath you, or use your hands to support your lower back. Roll your shoulders under and in toward your spine. Hold for 5 to 12 breaths.

4. To release, place your arms at your sides and lift your heels off the floor slightly as you draw your belly in and gradually lower your back down to the floor, starting at the top of your spine and rolling to the bottom. Your lower back should touch the floor before your buttocks do.

5. To provide a brief counterstretch, hug your knees to your chest, keeping your sacrum against the floor and your chin tucked slightly in, with your head still on the floor. Hold for 3 to 5 breaths, then lower one leg at a time back down to the floor and lie with your legs extended and arms by your sides. ◆

Tips: With each inhalation, lift your pelvis a bit higher.

— 8. BOTH-LEGS-UP RECLINE —

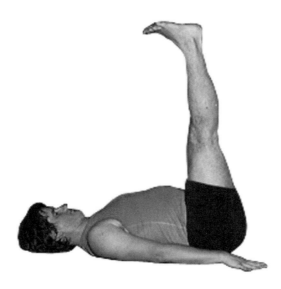

1. Still lying on your back with your arms by your sides and palms on the floor, exhale and bring your knees to your chest, keeping your sacrum pressed into the floor and your chin tucked slightly in.

2. As you inhale, extend your legs toward the ceiling while flexing your toes and feet toward your torso. Press your heels toward the ceiling. Hold for 5 to 12 breaths, keeping the small of your back on the floor throughout the pose.

3. To release, exhale, bend your legs, and hug your knees to your chest, keeping your sacrum against the floor and your chin tucked slightly in. Lower one leg at a time back down to the floor and lie with your legs extended and arms by your sides. ◆

Tips: You may also do this pose with your legs against a wall for support.

— 9. KNEE-DOWN TWIST —

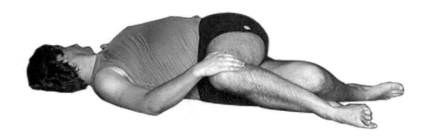

1. Still lying on your back, exhale and hug your knees to your chest with your knees touching each other.

2. Inhale and extend your arms out to the sides in line with your shoulders.

3. Exhale and lower your knees toward your right underarm while gazing over your left shoulder. Keep your abs contracted by drawing your belly in. You can use your right hand to gently press your left leg closer to the floor if you like. Hold for 5 to 12 breaths.

4. To release, inhale and return your knees to center, with your tailbone and lower back on the floor.

5. Keeping your knees to your chest, repeat steps 3 and 4 on the opposite side.

6. To finish, lower one leg at a time back down to the floor and lie with your legs extended and arms by your sides. ✦

Tips: Once you're in the pose, allow your legs to relax.

— 10. KNEES TO CHEST —

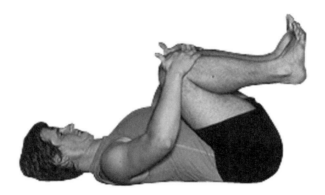

1. Still lying on your back, exhale and hug your knees to your chest. Keep your lower back on the floor and your chin tucked slightly in.

2. Work on pressing your sacrum to the floor as you hold for 3 to 5 breaths.

3. To release, lower one leg at a time back down to the floor and lie with your legs extended and arms by your sides. ✦

Tips: Think of the action as lengthening your lower back and spine, as opposed to pulling your knees closer to your chest.

— 11. RELAXATION POSE —

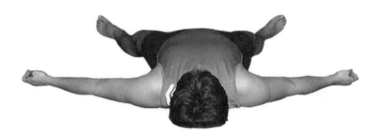

1. Still lying on your back, bring your legs out until your feet are a little farther than hip-width apart.

2. Take your arms out until they're at about a 30-degree angle from your sides, palms facing up. You may also rest your hands on your belly if you prefer.

3. Tuck your chin slightly into your chest while lengthening through the back of your head and neck.

4. Remain in this position for at least 5 minutes, letting your body relax as much as possible. Breathe naturally and make sure you always exhale slowly. ✦

Tips: If you feel strain in your lower back or if your low spine is overarching and rising off the floor, place a support such as a cushion or folded blanket under your knees.

Intermediate Practice Overview

Once you're comfortable with the beginner sequence, you can start working on the intermediate sequence below, which begins with a fluid and dynamic flow from one pose to the next, as in the sun salutations, in this case transitioning from Warrior 1 to Exalted Warrior. Start by learning the Strength Sun Salutation, earlier in the chapter. Because the poses in the core sequence, cooldown, and integration balance and build upon one another, it's best to do the entire sequence. However, if necessary it's fine to work on a few new poses from the intermediate core phase and cooldown and integration, below, during each session until you've learned all of them. As soon as you're ready, you can put the entire intermediate program together:

1. **Physical purification:** At a minimum, practice Uplifting Breath for 2 minutes and Calming Breath for 4 minutes, then do the Guided Body Scan and Relaxation for at least 5 minutes.

2. **Warm-up:** Do the complete warm-up sequence.

3. **Sun salutations:** Do at least three repetitions, including one or more Strength Sun Salutations.

4. **Intermediate sequence:** Do the core phase and cooldown and integration outlined below. In the core phase, anytime you return to Mountain at the end of a pose, you can pause for a breath or two to center yourself or rest before proceeding. Once you become very familiar with the full descriptions, you can use the sequence summary as a quick reference.

INTERMEDIATE SEQUENCE SUMMARY
INTERMEDIATE CORE PHASE —

1. Warrior 1 to Exalted Warrior to Side Lunge (4 times on each side, then to Mountain)

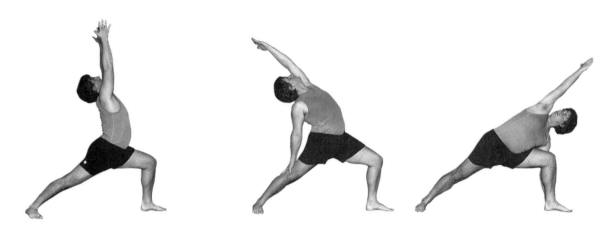

2. Hand to Big Toe (to Mountain)

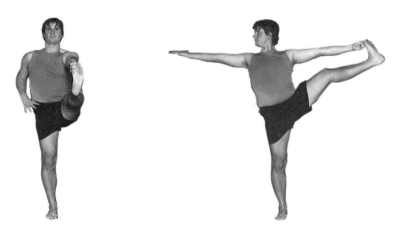

3. Dancer (to Mountain)

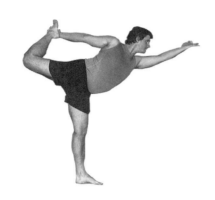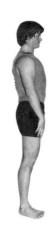

4. Half-Moon Leg Bent (to Mountain)

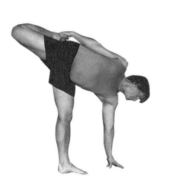

5. Reverse Triangle (to Mountain)

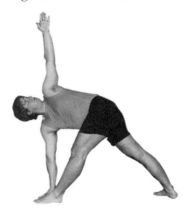

6. Goddess (to Mountain) ◆

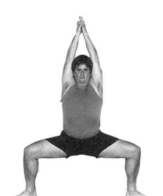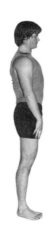

INTERMEDIATE COOLDOWN AND INTEGRATION —

1. Headstand (to Child's Pose)

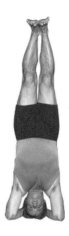

2. Shoulder Stand

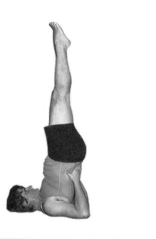

3. One-Leg-Down Shoulder Stand

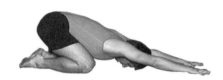

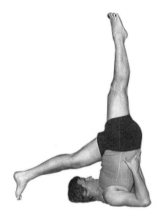

4. Modified Happy Baby

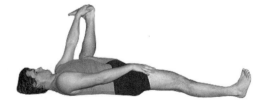

5. Full Wheel (to Knees to Chest)

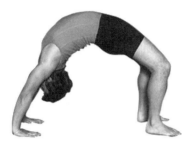 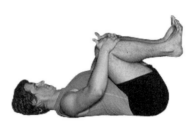

6. Knee-Down Twist

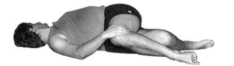

7. Relaxation Pose ✦

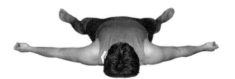

INTERMEDIATE CORE PHASE
— 1. WARRIOR 1 TO EXALTED WARRIOR TO SIDE LUNGE —

In this sequence, you start by doing Warrior 1, Exalted Warrior, and Side Lunge facing your left leg, or the front of the mat. First hold each pose for 5 to 12 breaths, then do 3 more repetitions of all three poses on that same side, holding each pose for just 1 breath. Then switch sides and repeat the entire sequence.

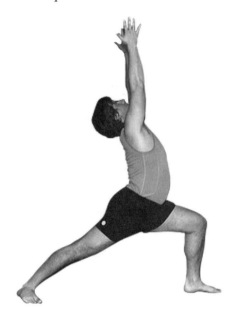

1. Begin in **Mountain**.

2. Inhale and step your right foot back. Your feet should be about the same distance apart as the length of one of your legs. Square your hips to the front of the mat and make sure your left foot is pointing toward the front of the mat. Exhale and turn your back foot slightly inward, toward your front heel.

3. Inhale and reach your arms overhead, palms facing each other, then exhale and bend your left leg, aligning the knee over your left ankle. Your leg should be bent to about 90 degrees. Hold for 5 to 12 breaths. (This is the pose **Warrior 1**.)

4. To transition to **Exalted Warrior**, inhale and slide your right hand down your right leg, avoiding putting extra weight onto the leg with your hand, then reach your left arm up and back as you rotate your chest up toward the ceiling. Hold for 5 to 12 breaths, then inhale and activate your core as you straighten your left leg and return to an upright position, gazing straight ahead.

5. To transition to **Side Lunge**, exhale and rotate your body 90 degrees to the right, keeping your left foot facing directly left and turning your right foot so that it's pointing slightly left, rather than directly toward the long side of the mat. Inhale and extend your arms to the sides at shoulder height, then exhale and bend your left leg, aligning the knee over your left ankle.

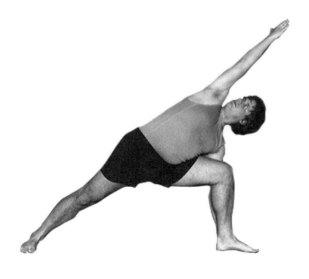

Exhale, lean to the left, keeping your spine long, and place your left hand on the floor close to the inside or outside of your left foot. Inhale and reach your right arm toward the ceiling or align it with the side of your body, reaching up and over your head. Hold for 5 to 12 breaths, then activate your core as you bring your torso upright with your arms at your sides.

6. Inhale, rotate 90 degrees to the left, with your left foot and your hips facing the front of the mat and your right foot turned so that it's pointing slightly left, rather than directly toward the long side of the mat, and come back to **Warrior 1** for 1 breath.

7. Inhale and return to **Exalted Warrior** for 1 breath.

8. Inhale and return to **Side Lunge** for 1 breath.

9. Repeat steps 6 through 8 twice more.

10. To transition to the other side, rotate 90 degrees to the right, with your right foot and your hips facing the back of the mat and your back foot pointing slightly right, rather than directly toward the long side of the mat.

11. Repeat steps 3 through 9 on the opposite side.

12. To finish, inhale and activate your core as you straighten your right leg and return to an upright position, gazing straight ahead and with your arms by your sides. Rotate 90 degrees to the left, with both feet and your hips pointing to the front of the mat, and step forward into **Mountain**. ✦

— 2. Hand to Big Toe —

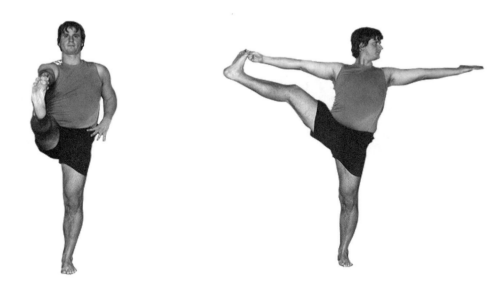

1. Beginning in **Mountain**, inhale and bend your right leg, bringing your knee toward your chest.

2. Grasp the big toe on your right foot with your index and middle fingers, exhale, and extend your right leg in front of you. Focus on lowering your right hip to keep it level with your left hip.

3. As you inhale, bring your right leg out to your right side, keeping it extended if possible. Hold for 5 to 12 breaths.

4. To release, inhale and return your right leg to center, keeping it raised and dropping your right hip again so it's level with your left hip. Release your grasp on your right foot, placing your hand on your right hip, and hold the leg extended to the front for 5 to 12 breaths.

5. Exhale and lower your leg, returning to **Mountain**. If necessary, pause in **Mountain** for a breath or two to recenter.

6. Repeat on the opposite side. ✦

Tips: If you need to, use a strap to help you straighten or hold your leg in the air. Initially, you may need to bend the raised leg to bring it to the side. As you gain strength and balance, work toward keeping it extended.

TRANSFORMATIVE YOGA

— 3. DANCER —

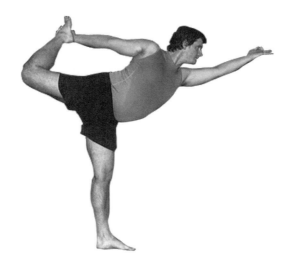

1. From **Mountain**, bend your right leg and lift your right foot off the floor behind you. Reach back and grab your right foot or ankle with your right hand. Flex your right foot.

2. As you inhale, reach your left arm out in front of you and slightly upward, palm facing up. Press your right foot into your right hand and lean forward, reaching out through your left arm. Hold for 5 to 12 breaths.

3. To release, exhale, let go of your right foot, and lower it to the floor alongside your left foot as you bring your body upright to return to **Mountain**.

4. Repeat on the opposite side. ◆

Tips: Each time you inhale, press your back foot into your hand to lift your leg slightly higher. Each time you exhale, extend your front arm a bit further forward as you open and lower your chest, but make sure your torso doesn't go lower than parallel to the ground.

— 4. HALF-MOON LEG BENT —

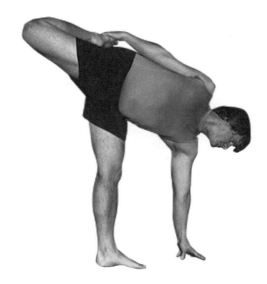

1. From **Mountain,** inhale and step your right foot back. Your feet should be about the same distance apart as the length of one of your legs.

2. Exhale and rotate your body 90 degrees to the right, keeping your left foot facing directly left and turning your right foot so that it's pointing slightly left, rather than directly toward the long side of the mat.

3. Inhale and extend your arms to the sides with your hands slightly higher than your shoulders.

4. As you exhale, bend sideways to the left, keeping your spine long, until your left hand touches your shin, ankle, or toes.

5. As you inhale, bend your left knee and lift your right foot off the floor. Bend your right knee and grasp your right foot with your right hand, rolling up through your lower ribs and chest. Gaze at the floor, or for a more challenging variation, gaze toward the ceiling. Hold for 5 to 12 breaths.

6. Each time you exhale, work to straighten the leg you're standing on, and each time you inhale, press your back foot into your hand as you roll your chest up toward the ceiling.

7. To release, bend your left leg slightly and lower your right foot to the floor beside your left foot. Exhale and come to **Standing Forward Bend**, relaxing your neck and back and bringing your chest and belly button toward your legs.

8. Inhale and return to an upright position, keeping your spine long and sweeping your arms up over your head, shoulder-distance apart, into **Extended Mountain**, with your back elongated in a gentle arch.

9. Exhale and return to **Mountain**, with your arms by your sides.

10. Repeat on the opposite side.

11. Turn around and come into **Mountain** at the front of your mat. ◆

Tips: For more of a challenge, extend your spine into a slight backbend.

— 5. REVERSE TRIANGLE —

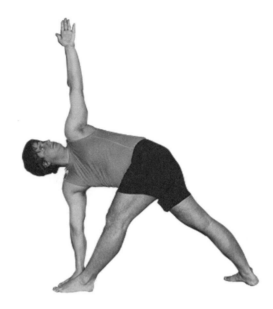

1. From **Mountain**, inhale and step your right foot back. Your feet should be about the same distance apart as the length of one of your legs, with your right leg turned slightly out. Draw your left hip back and push your right hip forward to maintain good alignment.

2. As you inhale, reach your right arm toward the ceiling.

3. As you exhale, hinge forward from the waist and place your right hand on the floor on either side of your left foot or on the foot.

4. Inhale and reach your left arm toward the ceiling as you twist your torso to the left. Hold for 5 to 12 breaths.

5. To release, exhale and come out of the twist, then inhale, contract the muscles in your right thigh, and activate your core as you straighten your left leg and gaze straight ahead.

6. Rotate your hips 180 degrees to the right, with your hips and right foot facing the right (the back of the mat) and your left foot turned slightly out. Repeat steps 2 through 5 on the opposite side.

7. Rotate your hips 180 degrees to the left, with your hips and feet facing the front of the mat, and step your right leg forward into **Mountain**. ✦

Tips: On each inhalation, deepen the twist while elongating your spine; think of lengthening out through the crown of your head.

— 6. GODDESS —

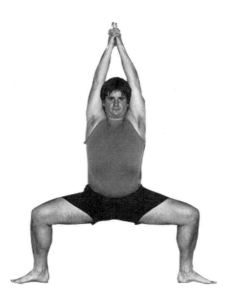

1. From **Mountain**, turn to face the long side of your mat, standing in the middle of the mat.

2. Inhale, step your right foot out about 3 feet to the side, then turn your feet out 90 degrees, so your toes point straight out to the ends of the mat.

3. Exhale and bend your knees to about 90 degrees, keeping your knees aligned over your ankles. Reach your arms over your head, placing your palms together, and pressing up through your index fingers.

4. Hold for 5 to 12 breaths, deepening into the pose each time you exhale.

5. To release, straighten your legs and bring your arms to your sides, then step your right foot back beside your left foot as you face the front of the mat. Rest and recenter in **Mountain** for 3 breaths before moving to the cooldown and integration. ✦

Tips: Lift your toes slightly away from the floor to protect your knees.

INTERMEDIATE COOLDOWN AND INTEGRATION

— 1. HEADSTAND —

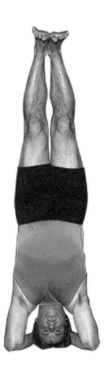

1. Begin on your hands and knees.

2. Bend your arms and bring your elbows to the floor, shoulder-distance apart. Grasp your elbows with your hands to ensure they're shoulder-distance apart, then place your forearms and wrists on the floor, creating a triangle shape, and interlace your fingers.

3. Bring the crown of your head to the floor, transferring your weight to your elbows and forearms as you do so.

4. Curl your toes under and lift your buttocks toward the ceiling.

5. Walk your feet toward your head until your hips are over your shoulders, keeping your elbows grounded to the floor.

6. Exhale and lift your legs off the floor, bending your knees and bringing them to your chest. Either stay in this position or straighten your legs, raising them toward the ceiling. Only attempt to straighten your legs if you can maintain and control the bent-knee headstand. Hold for up to 1 minute.

7. As you hold the position, contract your thigh muscles and touch your big toes together. Press further into your elbows and forearms; you'll feel your underarms begin to move slightly forward. Allow most of your weight to be on your arms and elbows. There will be some weight on your neck, but it shouldn't cause strain or discomfort in the neck.

8. To release, exhale and lower one leg at a time to the floor, then bring your buttocks to your heels and rest your forehead on the floor in **Child's Pose**, with your arms by your sides or stretched over your head with your palms on the floor. Hold for 5 breaths. ◆

Tips: Keep all of your movements steady to avoid neck strain, and make sure you're touching the crown of your head to the floor. Imagine **Headstand** as an upside-down version of **Mountain**, where your body is aligned from shoulder to hip, and through your ankles if your legs are extended. Your legs shouldn't swing up or down. Press up through the balls of your feet at the base of your big toes as you pull back through the outer edges of your feet toward your knees.

— 2. SHOULDER STAND —

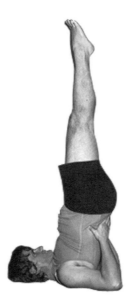

1. Lie on your back. Place your arms at your sides with your hands close to your hips.

2. As you exhale, lift your legs into the air, keeping them extended and keeping your sacrum on the floor.

3. As you inhale, press your palms into the floor and lift your tailbone up off the floor, then continue curling through your spine, extending your legs toward the ceiling as you bring your middle and upper back off the floor, and placing your hands on your back for support. Exhale.

4. Inhale and lift your legs toward the ceiling and extend your body, aligning your ankles over your hips and your hips over your shoulders. Rotate your legs inward a bit, press upward through the balls of your feet at the base of your big toes, and spread the rest of your toes.

5. Keep your chin in the center of your chest and gaze at your big toes. Hold for 2 minutes, breathing naturally, then continue to the next pose from this position. ◆

Tips: If you feel a lot of weight on the back of your neck, think of lengthening your legs further toward the ceiling and walk your elbows closer to each other. You can also lift your chin up and back to create more space in the back of your neck.

— 3. One-Leg-Down Shoulder Stand —

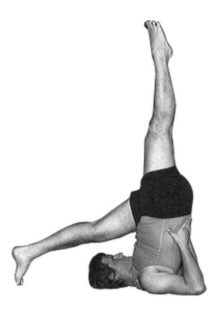

1. From **Shoulder Stand**, keep your left leg extended upward toward the ceiling as you exhale and slowly lower your right leg, keeping it extended, until the toes touch the floor over your head. Hold for 30 seconds, breathing naturally.

2. Inhale and slowly lift your right leg until you're once again in a full **Shoulder Stand**.

3. Repeat on the opposite side.

4. To release, bend your hips, allow your feet to extend slightly over your head, and return your palms to the floor beside your hips.

5. Exhale and roll down through your spine until your lower back and tailbone are on the floor, drawing your belly in to keep your abs tight.

6. Hug your knees to your chest, keeping your sacrum against the floor and your chin tucked slightly in. Hold for 1 breath, then lower one leg at a time back down to the floor and lie with your legs extended and arms by your sides. ✦

Tips: As you lower the leg to the floor, focus on keeping the other leg elongated toward the ceiling and engaged. This will help you maintain a long spine.

— 4. MODIFIED HAPPY BABY —

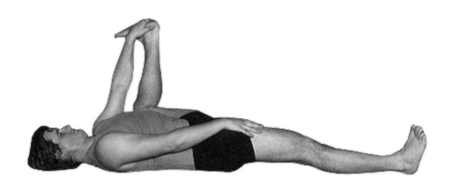

1. Still lying on your back, keep your left leg extended and on the floor as you exhale and bend your right leg, bringing your knee to your chest with your lower leg pointing straight up toward the ceiling. Grasp the sole of your right foot with your right hand.

2. Place your left hand on your left thigh, reaching toward your left knee, to help keep your left hip on the floor, then pull down on your right foot to press your right thigh toward the floor next to your rib cage. You can use your right upper arm to press your thigh toward the floor and deepen the stretch if you like, but don't press the leg down so far that your left hip rises.

3. Hold for 5 to 12 breaths.

4. To release, let go of your right foot and extend your right leg out on the floor alongside your left leg.

5. Repeat on the opposite side. ✦

Tips: Pull your bent leg downward while keeping the opposite leg as straight as you can.

— 5. FULL WHEEL —

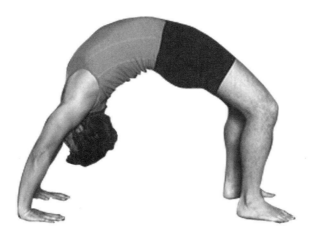

1. Still lying on your back, bend your legs and place your feet on the floor, hip-width apart and toes pointing straight ahead, with your heels as close to your buttocks as possible while keeping your pelvis on the floor.

2. Place your hands under your shoulders, elbows pointing toward the ceiling, with your palms down and your fingers pointing toward your feet.

3. As you inhale, press through your hands and feet, using your arms and legs to arch your back off the floor, with the top of your head touching the floor. Your elbows should be bent and about shoulder-distance apart, rather than splaying out. Exhale.

4. Inhale and straighten your arms, lifting your head off the floor and pressing through your feet as you arch your back. Hold for 5 to 12 breaths.

5. To release, bend your elbows and tuck your chin in as you lower your head to the floor, then gradually bring your upper back, then mid back, then lower back to the floor.

6. Hug your knees to your chest, keeping your sacrum against the floor and your chin tucked slightly in. Hold for 3 to 5 breaths, then lower one leg at a time back down to the floor and lie with your legs extended and arms by your sides. ◆

Tips: As you inhale, lift your chest and work to straighten your arms. As you exhale, draw your belly in to engage your core and maintain the position.

— 6. Knee-Down Twist —

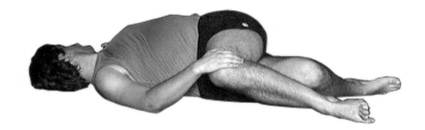

1. Still lying on your back, exhale and hug your knees to your chest with your knees touching each other. Inhale and extend your arms out to the sides in line with your shoulders.

2. Exhale and lower your knees toward your right underarm while gazing over your left shoulder. Keep your abs contracted by drawing your belly in. You can use your right hand to gently press your left leg closer to the floor if you like. Hold for 5 to 12 breaths.

3. To release, inhale and return your knees to center, with your tailbone and lower back on the floor.

4. Keeping your knees to your chest, repeat steps 2 and 3 on the opposite side.

5. To finish, lower one leg at a time back down to the floor and lie with your legs extended and arms by your sides. ✦

— 7. Relaxation Pose —

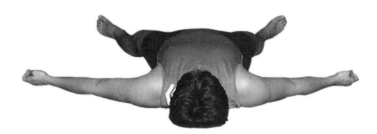

1. Still lying on your back, bring your legs out until your feet are a little wider than hip-width apart.

2. Take your arms out until they're at about a 30-degree angle from your sides, palms facing up. You may also rest your hands on your belly if you prefer.

3. Tuck your chin slightly into your chest while lengthening through the back of your neck.

4. Remain in this position for at least 5 minutes, letting your body relax as much as possible. Breathe naturally and make sure you always exhale slowly. ✦

Tips: If you feel strain in your lower back or if your low spine is overarching and rising off the floor, place a support such as a cushion or folded blanket under your knees.

Advanced Practice Overview

Once you're comfortable with the intermediate sequence, you can start working on the advanced sequence below. This practice is more advanced and incorporates fluid, dynamic transition through Downward Dog, using sequences from the sun salutations. Because the poses in the core sequence, cooldown, and integration balance and build upon one another, it's best to do the entire sequence. If necessary, however, it's fine to work on a few new poses from the advanced core phase and cooldown and integration during each session until you've learned all of them. As soon as you're ready, you can put the entire advanced program together:

1. **Physical purification:** At a minimum, practice Uplifting Breath for 2 minutes and Calming Breath for 4 minutes, then do the Guided Body Scan and Relaxation for at least 5 minutes.

2. **Warm-up:** Do the complete warm-up sequence.

3. **Sun salutations:** Do five repetitions of the Strength Sun Salutation.

4. **Advanced sequence:** Do the core phase and cooldown and integration outlined below. Once you become very familiar with the full descriptions, you can use the sequence summary as quick reference. ✦

Advanced Sequence Summary

Advanced Core Phase —

1. Warrior 2 to Side Lunge (6 times on each side)

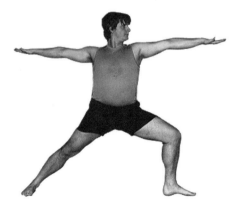 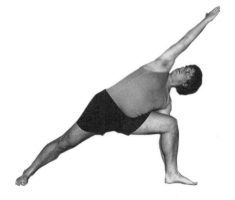

2. Transitioning Through Downward Dog

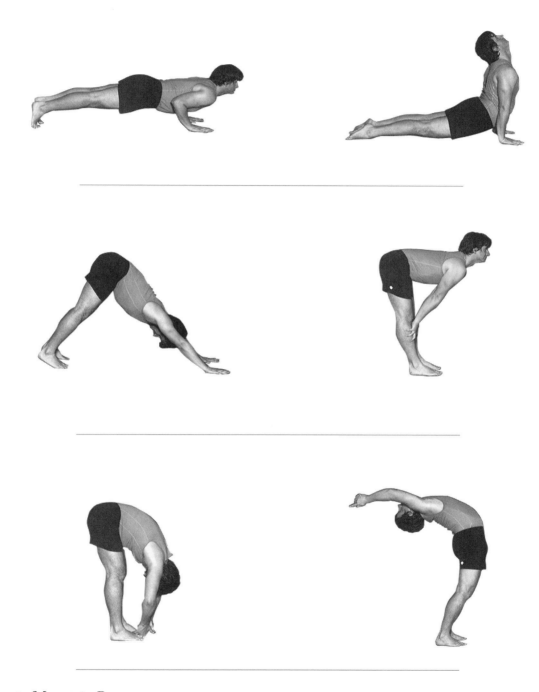

Return to Mountain Pose

3. Twisting Side Lunge

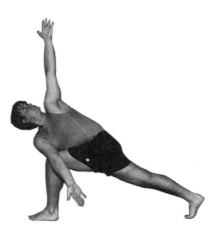

---

4. Transitioning Through Downward Dog

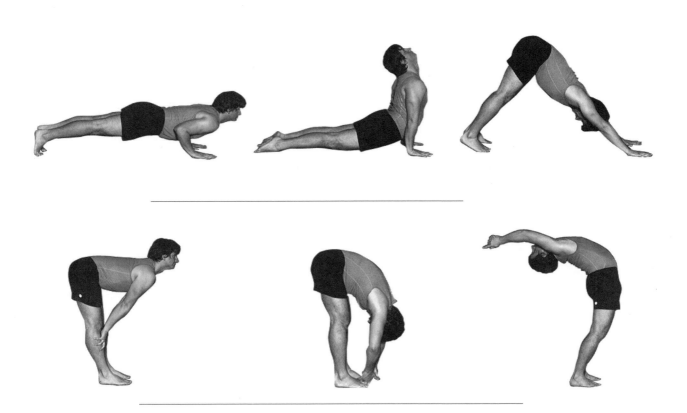

Return to Mountain Pose

5. Warrior 3

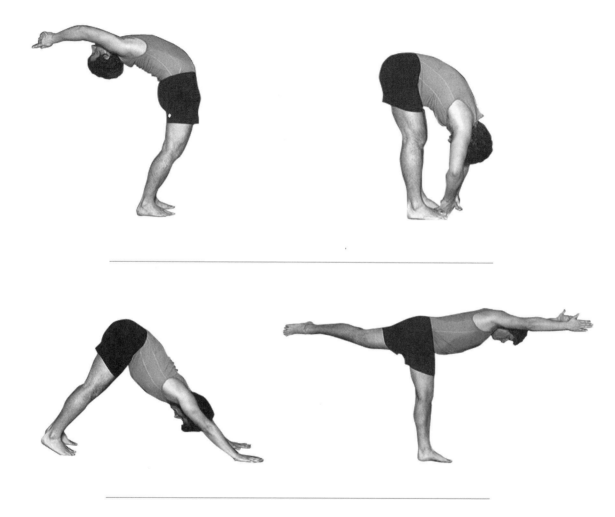

Return to Mountain Pose

6. Transitioning To Downward Dog

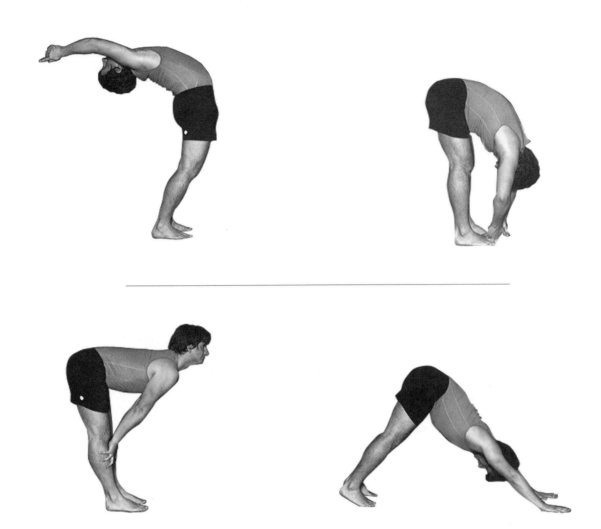

7. Side Crow to Flying Crow

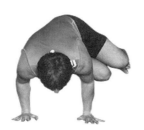

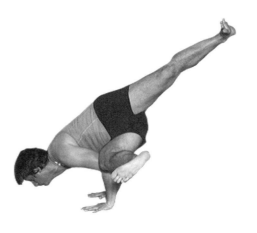

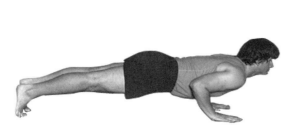

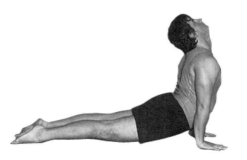

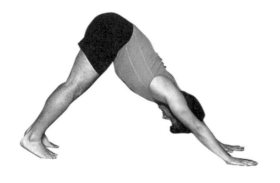

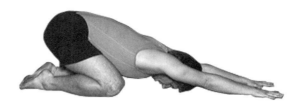

8. Forearm Balance

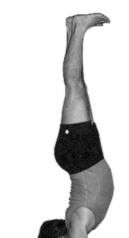

9. Headstand to Backbend

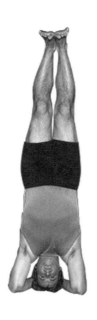
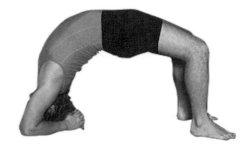

10. Full Wheel

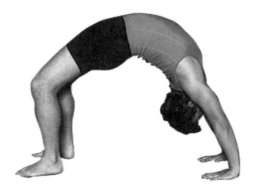

* Go to Child's Pose between each posture

11. Transitioning To Downward Dog

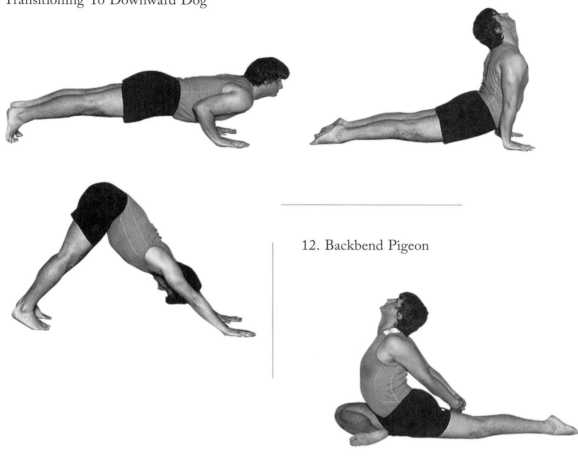

12. Backbend Pigeon

13. Camel

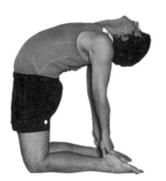

14. Downward Dog

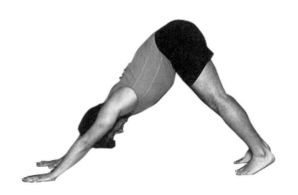

ADVANCED COOLDOWN AND INTEGRATION —

1. Seated Legs-Apart Forward Bend

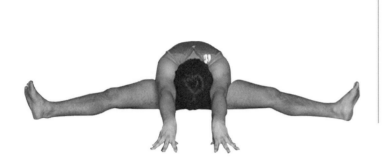

2. Hero

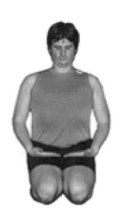

3. Twisting Hero

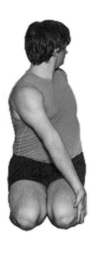

4. Shoulder Stand

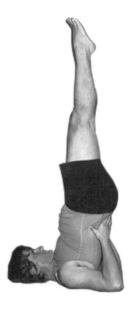

5. Plow (to Knees to Chest)

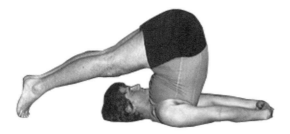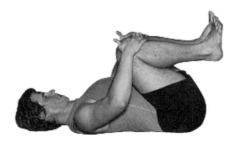

6. Supine Straight Legs to Side

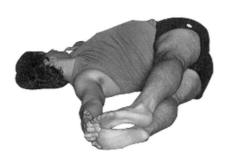

7. Relaxation Pose

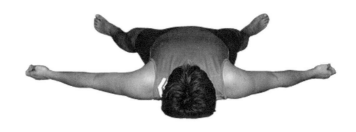

ADVANCED CORE PHASE

— 1. WARRIOR 2 TO SIDE LUNGE —

In this sequence, you start by doing Warrior 2 and Side Lunge with your left leg facing the front of the mat. First hold each pose for 5 to 12 breaths, then do 5 more repetitions on that same side, holding for each pose for just 1 breath. Then switch sides and repeat the entire sequence.

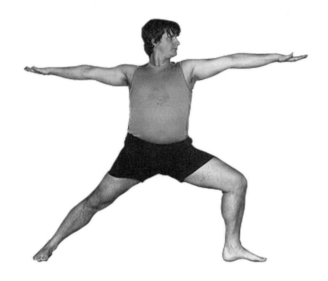

1. Begin in **Mountain**.

2. Inhale and step your right foot back. Your feet should be about the same distance apart as the length of one of your legs.

3. Exhale and rotate your body 90 degrees to the right, keeping your left foot facing directly left and turning your right foot 90 degrees, to point toward the long side of the mat.

4. Inhale and extend your arms to the sides at shoulder height, then exhale and bend your left leg, aligning your left knee over your left ankle. Your leg should be bent to about 90 degrees.

5. Gaze along your left arm, keeping your torso centered over your legs and your arms extended equally on either side. Lift your chest and drop your shoulders away from your ears. Lower your shoulder blades toward your hips. Hold for 5 to 12 breaths. (This is the pose **Warrior 2**.)

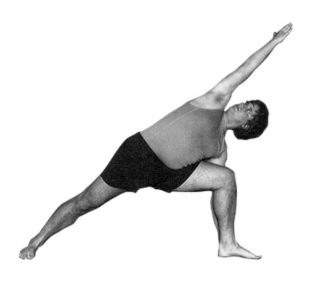

6. To transition to **Side Lunge**, exhale, lean to the left, keeping your spine long, and place your left hand on the floor close to the inside or outside of your left foot. Inhale and reach your right arm toward the ceiling or align it with the side of your body, reaching up and over your head. Hold for 5 to 12 breaths.

7. Inhale and come back to **Warrior 2** for 1 breath.

8. Exhale and move into **Side Lunge** for 1 breath.

9. Repeat steps 7 and 8 four more times.

10. To transition to the other side, inhale and activate your core as you straighten your left leg and return to an upright position, gazing straight ahead and with your arms by your sides. Rotate your left foot so that it's pointing slightly toward the right (back of the mat), rather than directly toward the long side of the mat, and turn your right foot directly to the right so it's pointing to the back of the mat.

11. Repeat steps 4 through 9 on the opposite side.

12. To finish, inhale and activate your core as you straighten your right leg and return to an upright position, gazing straight ahead and with your arms by your sides. Turn both feet toward the front of the mat and step into **Mountain** with your hips pointing to the front of the mat. ✦

— 2. TRANSITIONING THROUGH DOWNWARD DOG —

This transitional sequence is the same as the second half of the Strength Sun Salutation. Other transitional sequences in the Advanced Core Phase also make use of sequences from the sun salutations.

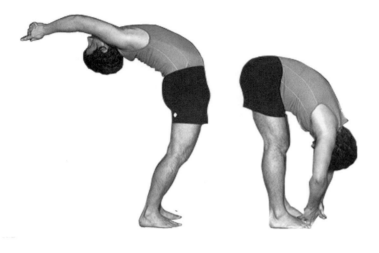

1. For the transition through **Downward Dog**, inhale and reach your arms up into **Extended Mountain**. Exhale and hinge forward from your hips, placing your hands on the floor shoulder-distance apart and on either side of both feet. Inhale and look halfway up.

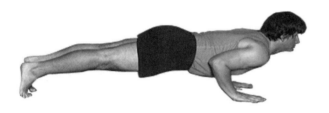

2. Exhale and step both feet back, keeping them hip-distance apart, and come into **Long Staff**, with your body in one straight line. Bend your elbows to lower your body a few inches above the ground and gaze forward, keeping your thigh muscles engaged and your belly in.

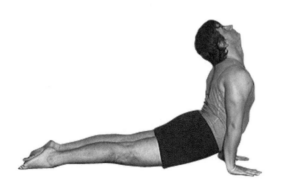

3. As you inhale, come into **Upward Dog** by lifting and pressing your chest forward and up, dropping your shoulder blades to keep your shoulders back and down, and keeping the tops of your toes and feet on the floor.

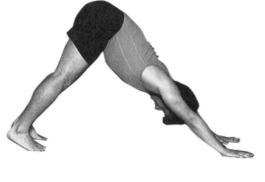

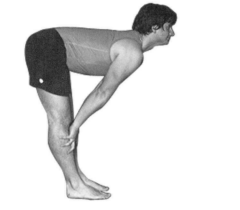

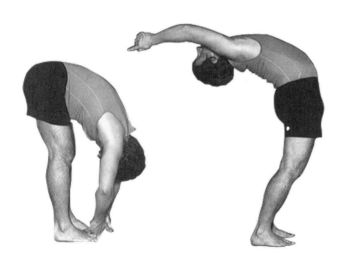

4. Exhale and come into **Downward Dog**, curling your toes under, then lifting your sit bones up toward the ceiling and straightening your legs. Keep your back long and gaze through your extended legs. Hold for 3 to 5 breaths.

5. Inhale and come into **Gazing Halfway Up**, stepping your feet up to a position between your hands, then straightening your legs, with your hands on the floor or on your ankles or shins, and gazing halfway up directly in front of you.

6. Exhale and come into **Standing Forward Bend**, relaxing your neck and back and bringing your chest and belly button toward your legs.

7. Inhale and come into **Extended Mountain**, hinging up and sweeping your arms up over your head, shoulder-distance apart, then extending back into a gentle arch.

8. Exhale and return to **Mountain**, with your arms by your sides. ✦

— 3. Twisting Side Lunge —

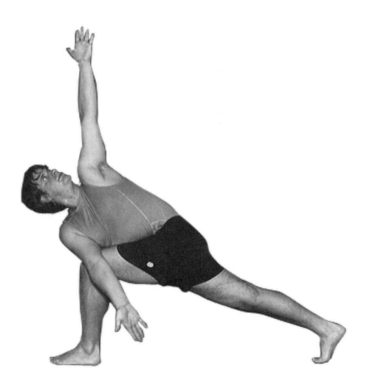

1. From **Mountain**, inhale and step your right foot back. Your feet should be about the same distance apart as the length of one of your legs, with your right leg turned slightly out. Draw your left hip back and push your right hip forward to maintain good alignment.

2. Exhale and bend your left leg, aligning the knee over your left ankle. Your leg should be bent to about 90 degrees. Maintain a strong connection with the outer edge of your right foot and heel.

3. Inhale and reach your right arm up.

4. As you exhale, lean forward and twist your torso to the left, keeping your spine long, and position your right elbow across your left knee. Bring your palms together, pointing your left elbow toward the ceiling.

5. Inhale, release your palms, and extend your arms, with your left hand pointing to the ceiling and your right hand pointing down toward the floor at an angle. Hold for 5 to 12 breaths.

6. To release, exhale and place your hands on floor as you come out of the twist. Inhale and activate your core as you straighten your left leg and bring your torso up. Gaze straight ahead, arms by your sides.

7. Rotate 180 degrees to the right, with your hips and right foot facing the right (the back of the mat) and your left foot turned slightly out. Repeat steps 2 through 6 on the opposite side.

8. Rotate 180 degrees to the left, with both of your feet and your hips facing the front of the mat. ◆

Tips: You may keep your back heel off the floor, or ground your heel, making sure that your back foot is slightly turned out.

— 4. Transitioning Through Downward Dog —

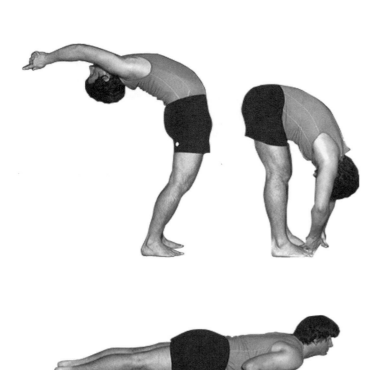

1. For the transition through **Downward Dog**, inhale and reach your arms up into **Extended Mountain**. Exhale and hinge forward from your hips, placing your hands on the floor shoulder-distance apart and on either side of both feet. Inhale and look halfway up.

2. Exhale and step both feet back, keeping them hip-distance apart, and come into **Long Staff**, with your body in one straight line. Bend your elbows to lower your body a few inches above the ground and gaze forward, keeping your thigh muscles engaged and your belly in.

3. As you inhale, come into **Upward Dog** by lifting and pressing your chest forward and up, dropping your shoulder blades to keep your shoulders back and down, and keeping the tops of your toes and feet on the floor.

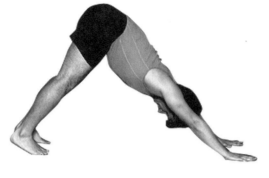

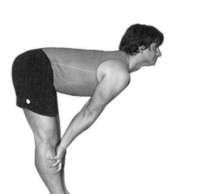

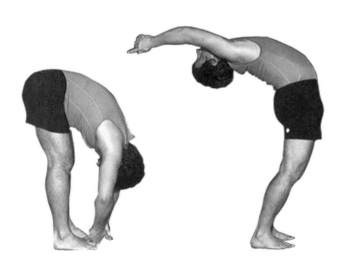

4. Exhale and come into **Downward Dog**, curling your toes under, then lifting your sit bones up toward the ceiling and straightening your legs. Keep your back long and gaze through your extended legs. Hold for 3 to 5 breaths.

5. Inhale and come into **Gazing Halfway Up**, stepping your feet up to a position between your hands, then straightening your legs, with your hands on the floor or on your ankles or shins, and gazing halfway up directly in front of you.

6. Exhale and come into **Standing Forward Bend**, relaxing your neck and back and bringing your chest and belly button toward your legs.

7. Inhale and come into **Extended Mountain**, hinging up and sweeping your arms up over your head, shoulder-distance apart, then extending back into a gentle arch.

8. Exhale and return to **Mountain**, with your arms by your sides. ✦

— 5. WARRIOR 3 —

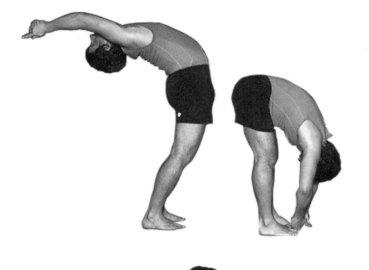

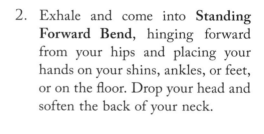

1. From **Mountain,** inhale and come into Extended Mountain, reaching your arms up over your head, shoulder-distance apart, and extending back into a gentle arch.

2. Exhale and come into **Standing Forward Bend,** hinging forward from your hips and placing your hands on your shins, ankles, or feet, or on the floor. Drop your head and soften the back of your neck.

3. Inhale and come into **Gazing Halfway Up,** gazing directly in front of you, elongating your spine, and working toward a slight arch.

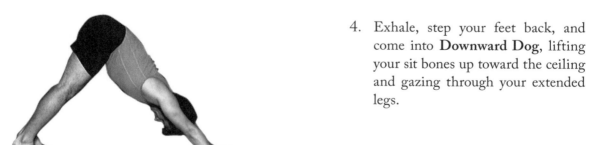

4. Exhale, step your feet back, and come into **Downward Dog,** lifting your sit bones up toward the ceiling and gazing through your extended legs.

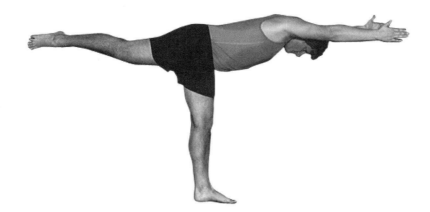

5. Put your weight in your right foot and lift your left leg back and up behind you.

6. Inhale and step your left foot up between your hands. Lift your right foot off the ground and straighten your left leg. Exhale and draw your belly in.

7. Inhale and reach both arms in front of you, holding them parallel to the floor at the same level as your shoulders, palms facing each other.

8. Gaze at the floor or through your extended arms and hold for 5 to 12 breaths.

9. To release, exhale and lower your hands to the floor as you lower your right foot to the floor beside your left foot. Bring your body upright to return to **Mountain**.

10. Repeat on the opposite side. ◆

Tips: Try to remain aligned from the foot that's off the floor to your fingertips, like a horizontal version of **Mountain**. With each inhalation, lengthen your body by extending through your arms and the lifted leg.

— 6. TRANSITIONING TO DOWNWARD DOG —

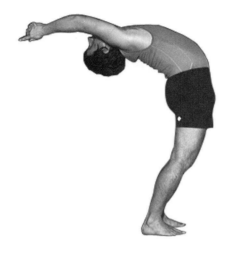

1. From **Mountain,** inhale and come into **Extended Mountain,** reaching your arms up over your head, shoulder-distance apart, and extending back into a gentle arch.

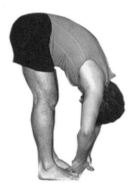

2. Exhale and come into **Standing Forward Bend,** hinging forward from your hips and placing your hands on your shins, ankles, or feet, or on the floor. Drop your head and soften the back of your neck.

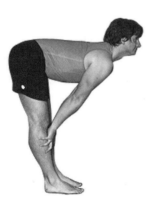

3. Inhale and come into **Gazing Halfway Up,** gazing directly in front of you, elongating your spine, and working toward a slight arch.

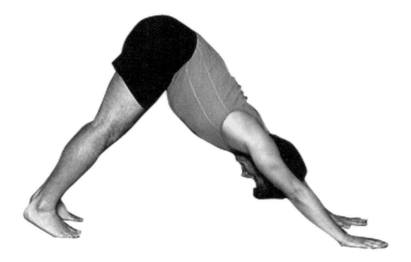

4. Exhale, step your feet back, and come into **Downward Dog,** lifting your sit bones up toward the ceiling and gazing through your extended legs. Hold for 3 to 5 breaths. ✦

— 7. SIDE CROW TO FLYING CROW —

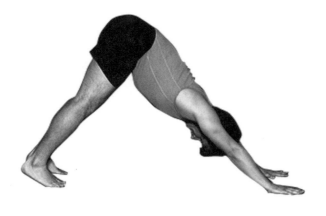

1. From **Downward Dog**, make sure your hands are shoulder-width apart, then walk your feet to the side of your left elbow.

2. Bend your arms and position the outside of your right knee on your left upper arm just above your left elbow, bending both of your legs and squeezing them together as you do so.

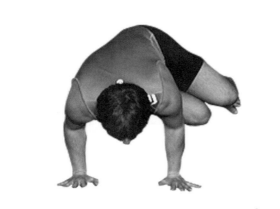

3. As you inhale, lean onto your hands, distributing your weight equally in both hands. Draw your belly in.

4. Lift your feet off the floor and draw your knees toward your ribs, pressing firmly through your hands and gazing at the ground between your hands. Hold for 3 to 5 breaths. (This is the pose **Side Crow**.)

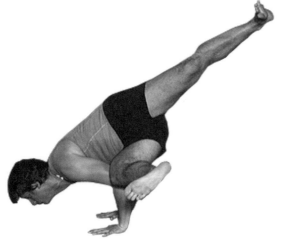

5. To transition into **Flying Crow**, begin to straighten your right leg out to the side while simultaneously extending your left leg back and up in line with the left side of your body. Hold for 5 to 12 breaths, being sure to keep your elbows by your sides, no more than shoulder-distance apart.

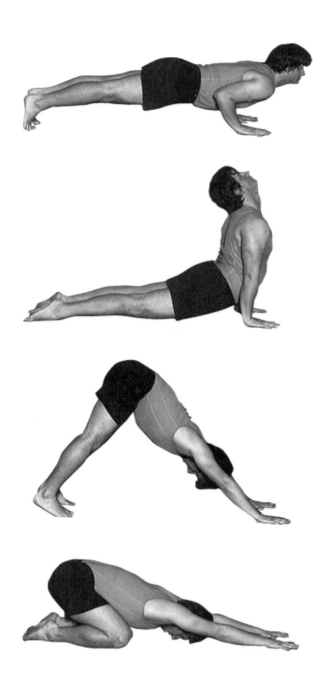

6. To release, exhale, bend your legs, and bring your knees back together. Lower your feet to the floor, then walk them back into **Long Staff**, with your body in one straight line. Bend your elbows, lowering your body a few inches above the ground, and gaze forward, keeping your thigh muscles engaged and your belly in.

7. Inhale and come into **Upward Dog** by lifting and pressing your chest forward and up, dropping your shoulder blades to keep your shoulders back and down, and keeping the tops of your toes and feet on the floor.

8. Exhale and come into **Downward Dog**, curling your toes under, then lifting your sit bones up toward the ceiling and straightening your legs. Keep your back long and gaze through your extended legs.

9. Bend your knees and come to an all-fours position, then bring your buttocks to your heels and rest your forehead on the floor in **Child's Pose**, with your arms by your sides or stretched over your head. Hold for 3 to 5 breaths.

10. Repeat on the opposite side. ✦

Tips: Use weight transference to come into the pose, rather than relying mostly on your arms and shoulders.

— 8. Forearm Balance —

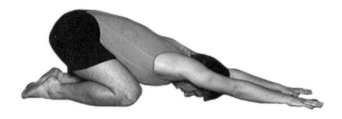

1. From **Child's Pose** come to an all-fours position, then bend your arms and bring your elbows to the floor, shoulder-distance apart.

2. Place your forearms and wrists on the floor. Your forearms should be right in front of your elbows.

3. Curl your toes under and lift your buttocks toward the ceiling.

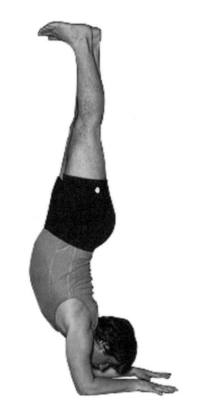

4. Walk your feet toward your elbows, maintaining the connection to the floor through your elbows and transferring your weight to your forearms.

5. Inhale and bring one leg at a time up directly over your shoulders.

6. Gaze at the floor between your hands and hold for up to 1 minute.

7. To release, keep your belly in as you return one leg at a time to the floor with a controlled motion, then come to an all-fours position.

8. From the all-fours position with your big toes touching, exhale, bring your buttocks to your heels, and allow your forehead to rest on the floor in **Child's Pose**. Place your arms by your sides or stretch them over your head with your palms on the floor. Hold for 5 to 12 breaths. ✦

Tips: To help with balance, reach your legs upward and keep the thigh muscles engaged for stronger core awareness. A steady gaze will also help you stay balanced.

— 9. HEADSTAND TO BACKBEND —

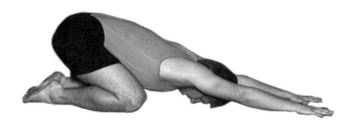

1. From **Child's Pose**, come onto all fours and place your elbows on the floor, shoulder-distance apart. Grasp your elbows with your hands to ensure they're shoulder-distance apart, then place your forearms and wrists on the floor, creating a triangle shape, and interlace your fingers.

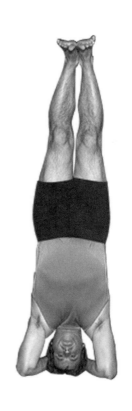

2. Bring the crown of your head to the floor between your hands, transferring your weight to your elbows and forearms as you do so.

3. Curl your toes under and lift your buttocks toward the ceiling.

4. Walk your feet toward your head until your hips are over your shoulders, keeping your elbows grounded to the floor.

5. Exhale and lift your legs off the floor, bending your knees and bringing them to your chest. Straighten your legs, raising them toward the ceiling, and hold for up to 2 minutes.

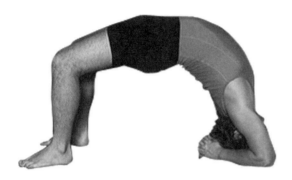

6. As you hold the position, contract your thigh muscles and touch your big toes together. Press further into your elbows and forearms; you'll feel your underarms begin to move slightly forward. Allow most of your weight to be on your arms and elbows. There will be some weight on your neck, but it shouldn't cause strain or discomfort in the neck.

7. To transition into **Backbend**, soften your back and press your ribs forward slightly.

8. Take one leg over your head until the foot touches the floor, quickly followed by the other leg. Your forearms and elbows should still be on the floor at this point. ✦

Tips: As you bring each leg over your head to the floor, keep your shoulders strong and the back of your body soft; move slowly and remain calm.

— 10. Full Wheel —

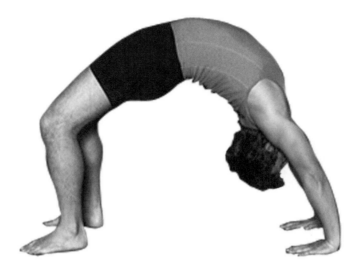

1. From **Backbend,** release your hands and position your palms on the floor, shoulder-distance apart.

2. Inhale and straighten your arms, lifting your head off the floor and pressing through your feet as you extend your spine and increase the arch. Hold for 5 to 12 breaths.

3. To release, bend your elbows and tuck your chin in as you lower your head to the floor, then gradually bring your upper back, then mid back, then lower back to the floor.

4. Hug your knees to your chest, keeping your sacrum against the floor and your chin tucked slightly in. Hold for 3 to 5 breaths, then lower one leg at a time back down to the floor and lie with your legs extended and arms by your sides. ◆

— 11. Transitioning to Downward Dog —

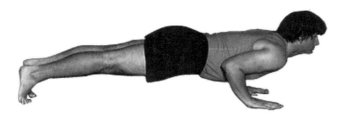

1. To transition into **Downward Dog**, hug your knees to your chest, then roll up to a cross-legged position. Put your palms on the floor in front of you, shoulder-distance apart, and jump or step your feet back into **Long Staff**, with your body in one straight line. Bend your elbows to lower your body a few inches above the ground and gaze forward, keeping your thigh muscles engaged and your belly in.

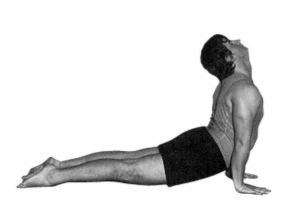

2. As you inhale, come into **Upward Dog** by lifting and pressing your chest forward and up, dropping your shoulder blades to keep your shoulders back and down, and keeping the tops of your toes and feet on the floor.

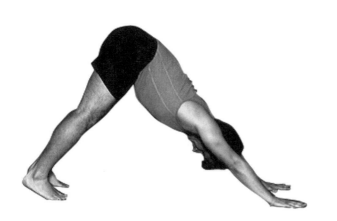

3. Exhale and come into **Downward Dog**, curling your toes under, then lifting your sit bones up toward the ceiling and straightening your legs. Keep your back long and gaze through your extended legs. Hold for 1 breath. ✦

— 12. BACKBEND PIGEON —

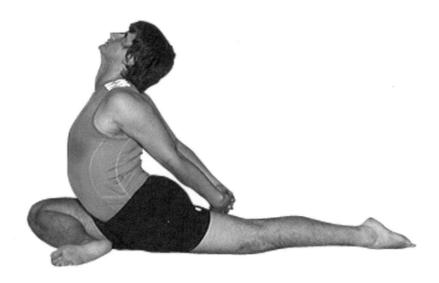

1. From **Downward Dog**, come to an all-fours position. Bring your right knee forward to a position just inside your right hand, angling your lower leg toward the left so you rest on the outside of your right shin. If you look down, your right leg should be bent about 20 to 30 degrees.

2. Point your hips squarely toward the floor as you extend your left leg behind you, with the top of the foot and knee touching the floor.

3. Reach your hands behind your back, interlace your fingers, and extend your arms. As you inhale, lift your chest and roll your shoulders back and down. Hold for 5 to 12 breaths.

4. To release, exhale and place your hands on the floor on either side of your right knee, shoulder-distance apart, and return to the all-fours position.

5. Repeat on the opposite side. ✦

Tips: Draw your belly in and keep the hip bone on the leg that's extended behind you sinking and pointing down to the floor to align with the other hip.

— 13. CAMEL —

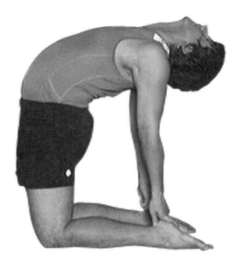

1. From the all-fours position, come up to a kneeling position, with your body upright and your shins and the tops of your feet on the floor.

2. Place your palms on your back, fingers pointing down, to support your lower back and sacrum.

3. Inhale and press your hands into your lower back to push your hips forward as you elongate your spine and lift your chest up and away from your belly button toward the ceiling, extending back into a **Backbend**. Keep your hips aligned with your knees.

4. Slide your hands down then reach them back, one at a time, to grasp your heels. Keep your chin in or let your head tilt all the way back, keeping your neck elongated. Hold for 5 to 12 breaths.

5. To release, come up to a kneeling position, rolling one shoulder up at a time. Return to the all-fours position. ✦

Tips: Keep your hips pointing forward and aligned over your knees to avoid back strain. With each inhalation, lengthen through the front of your body as you lift your chest. With each exhalation press your hips forward to maintain good alignment, with your hips over your knees.

— 14. Downward Dog —

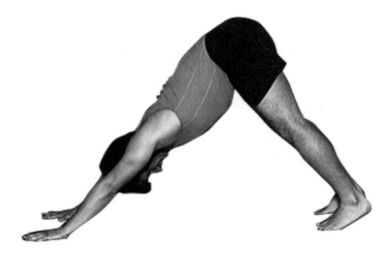

1. Still in the all-fours position, make sure your knees and feet are about hip-width apart.

2. Keeping your palms firmly on the floor, curl your toes under, then exhale and lift your sit bones toward the ceiling, straightening your legs.

3. Gaze through your extended legs and spread your fingers and toes wide. Press through the balls of your feet at the base of your big toes and through your thumbs and index fingers.

4. Hold for 3 to 5 breaths.

5. To release, exhale, jump or walk your legs through your hands, and come to a seated position with your legs extended in front. ✦

— 1. SEATED LEGS-APART FORWARD BEND —

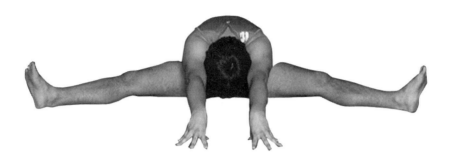

1. Still sitting with your legs extended in front of you, bring your legs wide apart, keeping them on the floor and extended. Your knees should be pointed directly toward the ceiling.

2. Place your hands on the floor behind your back, inhale, and straighten your arms to lengthen your spine.

3. Exhale and hinge forward, keeping your thigh muscles contracted and sliding your hands out directly in front of you. Only go as far as you can without rounding through your mid and upper back. Hold for 5 to 12 breaths.

4. To release, inhale, walk your hands up toward your pelvis, and bring your torso back upright. Reach one hand under one knee and bend the leg, then do the same thing with the other leg. One at a time, bring your legs to a cross-legged position for 1 breath. ✦

Tips: Keep your sit bones on the ground and your chest lifted as you lean forward. Press out through the balls of your feet at the base of your big toes.

— 2. HERO —

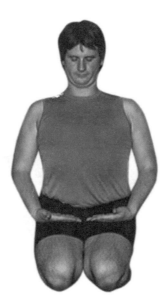

1. Sit on your heels with your knees and thighs touching and drawn toward each other.

2. Inhale and elongate through your spine, then roll your shoulders up to your ears, then exhale and continue rolling your shoulders until they're back and down.

3. Rest the backs of your hands on your thighs, fingertips pointing toward one another and tuck your chin down slightly. Hold for 3 to 5 breaths, then continue to **Twisting Hero** from this position. ◆

Tips: Lift and open the center of your chest and avoid slouching. Use a folded blanket or yoga block under your buttocks if you feel tension in your knees, or to protect your knees if you sit in this posture for a long time, such as during meditation.

— 3. TWISTING HERO —

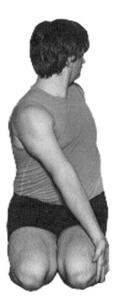

1. From **Hero,** inhale and place your right hand on the outside of your left knee or thigh. Extend your left arm behind you a bit higher than the level of your shoulder or put your left palm on your lower back.

2. Exhale and look over your left shoulder, making sure your hips remain level and square to the front. Hold for 5 to 12 breaths.

3. To release, inhale and return to gazing straight ahead and place your hand on your thighs.

4. Repeat on the opposite side. ◆

Tips: Keep your spine long and twist from the middle of your back. If you feel any tension in your knees, place a folded blanket or yoga block between your heels and buttocks. Keep your knees and thighs hugging toward the midline of your body throughout the movement.

— 4. SHOULDER STAND —

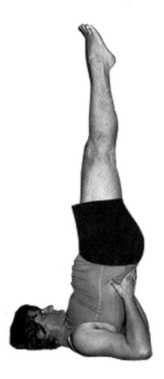

1. Lie on your back. Place your arms at your sides with your hands close to your hips.

2. As you exhale, lift your legs into the air, keeping them extended and keeping your sacrum on the floor.

3. As you inhale, press your palms into the floor and lift your tailbone up off the floor, then continue curling through your spine, extending your legs toward the ceiling as you bring your middle and upper back off the floor, and placing your hands on your back for support.

4. Inhale and lift your legs toward the ceiling and extend your body, aligning your ankles over your hips and your hips over your shoulders. Rotate your thighs inward and press upward through the balls of your feet at the base of your big toes, keeping the rest of your toes spread.

5. Keep your chin in the center of your chest and gaze at your big toes. Hold for 3 minutes, breathing naturally, then continue to **Plow** from this position. ◆

— 5. Plow —

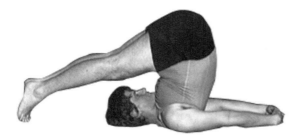 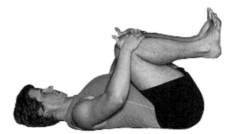

1. From **Shoulder Stand**, exhale and slowly lower your feet over your head, keeping your legs extended, bringing your feet to the floor with your toes curled under.

2. You may keep your hands on your lower back; lower them to the floor, extending your arms and placing your palms on the floor shoulder-distance apart; or interlace your fingers and lower your hands to the floor, extending your arms.

3. Hold for 1 minute, keeping your hips aligned over your shoulders. Hold your chin in the center of your chest and keep your spine long.

4. To come out of the pose, return your hands to your back for support, then extend your legs in the air so you're back in a **Shoulder Stand,** then exhale and roll down through your spine until your lower back and tailbone are on the floor, drawing your belly in to keep your abs tight.

5. Hug your knees to your chest, keeping your sacrum against the floor and your chin tucked slightly in. Hold for 3 to 5 breaths, then lower one leg at a time back down to the floor and lie with your legs extended and arms by your sides. ✦

Tips: For proper alignment of your hips over your shoulders and to avoid rounding your spine, keep your toes curled under and walk your feet slightly toward your head.

— 6. SUPINE STRAIGHT LEGS TO SIDE —

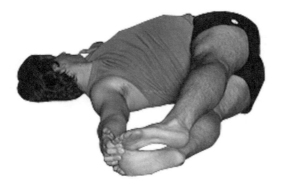

1. Still lying on your back, exhale and bring your extended legs up to 90 degrees, pressing into your palms to help with the lifting motion and keeping your tailbone pressed against the floor.

2. Inhale and extend your arms out to the sides in line with your shoulders.

3. Exhale and lower your legs to the floor on your right side, keeping your legs straight and your shoulders as grounded as you can, keeping your left shoulder working toward the floor.

4. Gaze over your left shoulder and hold for 5 to 12 breaths, allowing your legs to fully relax.

5. To release, inhale and return your legs back to the center, until your legs are extended straight up and your tailbone is grounded once again.

6. Repeat on the opposite side.

7. To finish, lower one leg at a time back down to the floor and lie with your legs extended and arms by your sides. ✦

Tips: Use your exhalation to deepen into the posture. If this is difficult or strains your lower back, you can bend your knees.

— 7. Relaxation Pose —

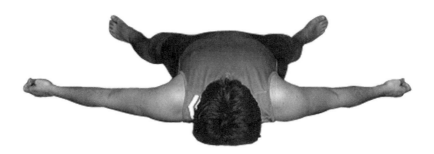

1. Still lying on your back, bring your legs out until your feet are a little farther than hip-width apart.

2. Take your arms out until they're at about a 30-degree angle from your sides, palms facing up. You may also rest your hands on your belly if you prefer.

3. Tuck your chin slightly into your chest while lengthening through the back of your head and neck.

4. Remain in this position for at least 5 minutes, letting your body relax as much as possible. Breathe naturally and make sure you always exhale slowly. ◆

YOUR YOGA JOURNEY CONTINUES

Spend time practicing the movements in this chapter in the sequences shown. Only with practice can you improve your technique and eventually advance to more complex postures. However, it isn't necessary to master all of the postures in this chapter before moving on to chapter 2. What is important is to engage in regular practice. Once you get a feel for how yoga can benefit you on a physical level, it's time to take the next step in your journey toward profound inner peace.

CHAPTER 2

ENERGY

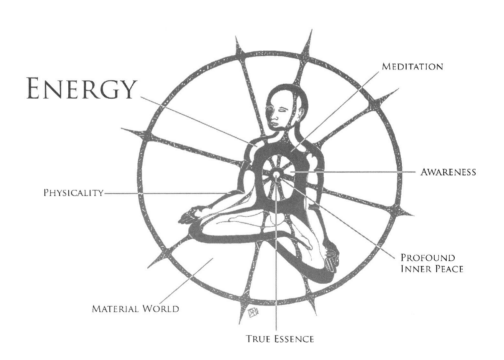

ENERGY

MEDITATION

AWARENESS

PHYSICALITY

PROFOUND
INNER PEACE

MATERIAL WORLD

TRUE ESSENCE

Everything in life is propelled by energy. Energy—or prana as it's called in yoga—is your life force. It's the focus of the second kosha, discussed in this chapter. In order for your physical body to thrive, and even be alive, prana must be present. You can't see this energy, but you can get a sense of how it works by focusing on your breathing. Breath is the transporter of prana. As you breathe in, you draw prana through your body. As you breathe out, prana leaves your body, taking toxins with it.

When your breathing is full and relaxed, such as during yogic breathing through your nose, energy flows freely through your body. This is a sign of a healthy second kosha—your energy kosha. On the other hand, when you're stressed-out your breathing tends to be quick and shallow, which inhibits a proper flow of energy and suggests that your energy kosha could use some attention.

So if prana is your life force and you need to breathe to stay alive, are breath and energy one and the same? No. They're highly connected but distinct from one another. Breath is not energy. Breath is not prana. Breath is the *vehicle* for energy. Here's another way to look at it: Your breath is the lens you use to see how your prana is doing. Because the integrity of your prana is reflected in your breath, calm, purposeful, and, most importantly, conscious breathing equals a good flow of energy, which indicates a healthy energy kosha.

LETTING ENERGY FLOW

In this chapter, you'll explore how you are more than just your physical body and consider the internal nature of your kosha layers. In doing so, you'll begin to strengthen the communication between your body and your mind, building on a framework of conscious breathing and kosha philosophy. Just as you're able to revitalize physical health through the physical practice of yoga, you can nurture healthy koshas and a strong flow of energy within yourself through a combination of postures and breathwork.

When you feel physically energetic, perhaps from good nutrition and healthful living, you're better able to perform yoga postures, get up in the morning, do your work effectively, and simply move around each day. And just as physical energy uplifts your body, energy in the form of prana uplifts your inner being, allowing you to connect to higher places within your consciousness. When your energy is stagnant and unhealthy, on the other hand, you'll probably struggle to tap into your more subtle koshas as a way to gain awareness and deeper insight about your true self.

Energy naturally courses throughout the body, but it can also be focused and directed toward certain areas. The following pages contain guidelines for accessing and experimenting with various energy flows. You'll learn how to channel your breath to five areas of your body for the purpose of heightened consciousness and a more purified energy kosha. There are numerous internal energy flows, but the five you'll focus on are especially recommended for supporting the practice of yoga and the kosha philosophy. For the purposes of this book, these five energy flows are referred to as grounding, core, clarity, vitality, and wholeness:

1. **Grounding:** Energy in the legs
2. **Core:** Energy directed to the body's center
3. **Clarity:** Energy in the head
4. **Vitality:** Energy flowing from the navel to the heart
5. **Wholeness:** Energy radiating from the belly to every extremity

As you journey into this exploration of energetics, you'll begin to discover and hopefully feel the movement of these pranic currents in your body. This is an indication that your energy kosha is becoming stronger. The goal here is to understand on a deeper level how the practice of asanas is ultimately not about how flexible you are or how far you can bend. It's about cultivating a relationship with and awareness of your energy as a vital kosha layer, then harnessing, guiding, and controlling that energy to your yogic advantage. That in itself sounds like a monumental task, but as this chapter progresses you'll see how to successfully unleash the power of prana through asanas and breathing exercises.

As you move forward, create an intention to achieve a more balanced state for yourself—a state that is grounded and alert at the same time. Through the movement sequences and conscious breathing exercises described in this chapter, you'll revitalize your energy kosha, resulting in greater vitality, awareness, and mental clarity.

FIVE PRACTICES FOR REVITALIZING YOUR ENERGY KOSHA

What's Your Energetic State?

This chapter offers five sequences of postures. Each one cultivates or complements a different energetic state, but you can also practice all five in one session if you like. To determine which practice might benefit you most at any given time, ask yourself this simple question: How do I feel?

- If you feel anxious, restless, overstimulated, or buzzed out on caffeine, choose the Grounding or Core Sequence.

- If you feel tired, lethargic, or heavy, choose the Clarity or Vitality Sequence.

- If you feel balanced, stable, or clearheaded, choose the Wholeness Sequence.

In chapter 1, you became acquainted with the physicality of yoga through a series of poses at three levels: beginner, intermediate, and advanced. In this chapter, you'll continue your asana practice, but now it's time to focus a little more inward. You'll turn your attention to conscious movement and ujjayi breathwork as a way to get in touch with your internal energy currents and prepare for the meditation practices in later chapters. These techniques will help you create a healthier relationship with your energy kosha.

The posture sequences and breathing exercises presented in this chapter are brief. You can complete each one in about 20 minutes, including the warm-up. Choose one or all five. You may also continue doing sequences from chapter 1. Here are some guidelines to keep in mind as you do the work in this chapter:

- Refer to the text box "What's Your Energetic State?" to determine the right energy-stimulating sequences for your present disposition.

- Begin all of the sequences in this chapter with two repetitions of the Strength Sun Salutation as a warm-up.

- End each session with the Three-Seal Breathing technique described on page 132.

Energy-stimulating sequences are best done in the afternoon simply because they involve forward bends and backbends, which tend to be easier to accomplish once you've limbered up from moving around during your day. However, almost any time of day is fine, and it's better to fit this practice in whenever you can than not do it at all. Just avoid doing these routines too close to bedtime, as they may overstimulate your nervous system when you should be settling down for the night. Complete any energy-stimulating sequence at least two hours before you plan to go to bed.

Strength Sun Salutation Warm-Up —

A proper warm-up increases heat in the body and lubricates your joints. To avoid injury and enhance your yoga practice, perform the following Strength Sun Salutation two times as a warm-up before doing any of the energy-stimulating sequences in this chapter. By now you're probably familiar with the Strength Sun Salutation, but if you need a refresher on any of the particulars, refer back to chapter 1 for a full description.

1. Mountain

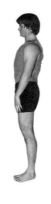

2. Extended Mountain

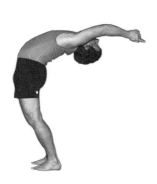

3. Standing Forward Bend

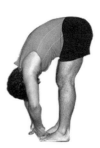

4. Gazing Halfway Up

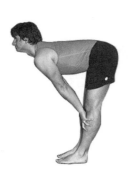

5. Long Staff

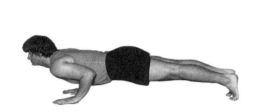

6. Upward Dog

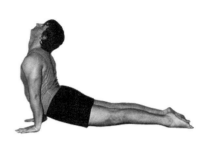

7. Downward Dog

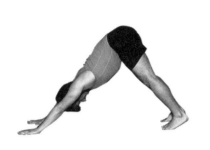

8. Gazing Halfway Up

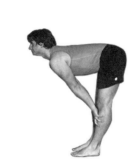

9. Standing Forward Bend

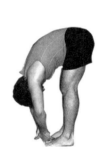

10. Extended Mountain

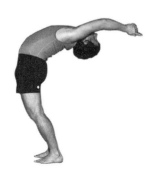

11. Mountain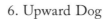

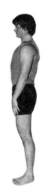

STRENGTH SUN SALUTATION

— THREE-SEAL BREATHING —

The purpose of Three-Seal Breathing is to hold energy, or prana, in the body. This breathing technique guides prana toward your spine, then upward to your brain, where it stimulates the third eye chakra, which is the seat of consciousness. When the third eye is stimulated, it allows for greater awareness and a heightening of the senses. The three seals that hold energy within the body are the root seal, the chin seal, and the navel seal: The root seal involves contracting your perineum by squeezing your anal sphincter. The chin seal involves tucking your chin 20 degrees down toward your throat. The navel seal involves drawing your belly in and up as if scooping under your rib cage.

Here are complete instructions for Three-Seal Breathing. Follow this procedure once, at the end of your practice of energy sequences. If you do multiple energy sequences, just do the Three-Seal Breathing once, at the end of all energy sequences:

1. Sit in a comfortable cross-legged position on the floor with your spine long or sit in a chair with the back of the chair supporting your back. (If you sit cross-legged, remember to ensure that your knees are below the top of your hip bones. If necessary, sit on a cushion or yoga bolster to achieve this position.)

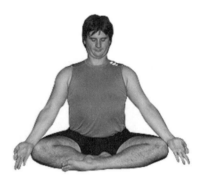

2. Close your eyes. Breathe in and out through your nose.

3. As you inhale, contract your perineum by squeezing your anal sphincter. This is the root seal.

4. At the end of your inhale, draw your chin down 20 degrees and retract your head slightly so your ears align over your shoulders. This is the chin seal.

5. As you exhale, maintain both the root seal and the chin seal.

6. At the end of your exhalation, rapidly draw your belly in and up. This is the navel seal.

7. Inhale and release all three seals. Exhale naturally. ✦

ENERGY FLOW: GROUNDING

Each energy flow corresponds to one of nature's elements, and it's not surprising that energy flowing through your legs represents earth. Feeling down-to-earth or grounded involves a strong connection with your physical body. Hopefully you've begun to cultivate that through your yoga practice from chapter 1.

Getting in touch with your grounding energy is especially important in modern life. Think of how you go about your day. A lot of your activities are probably focused around your head, neck, shoulders, and arms: clutching your car's steering wheel, taking phone calls, plugging into an MP3 player, typing e-mails, and so on. You can balance all that busyness in the upper body with postures and breathing techniques that pull your energy toward the earth for a more rooted sense of self.

When you're in a grounded state, you're more likely to experience feelings of serenity and calmness because your thinking is clearer; basically, your head isn't in the clouds. The brain can't be calm if grounding energy is inhibited. Healthy downward energy allows you to experience the present—be in the moment—with greater ease. When your conscious self is rooted in the here and now, inward reflection can begin to occur. For example, if your mind is busy worrying about what happened at work yesterday or what's for dinner five hours from now, you won't be able to set the stage for meditation. Grounding energy anchors the mind and body so true meditation comes more readily.

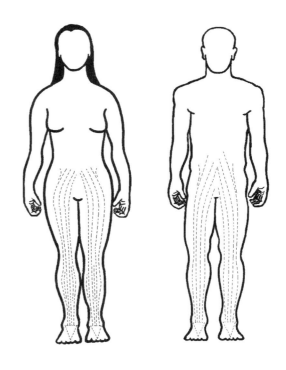

GROUNDING SEQUENCE

Just as grounding energy roots you mentally, some postures root you physically by stabilizing your body or encouraging a downward flow of energy. Even just touching your bare feet to the floor or a yoga mat encourages a greater connection to the earth, and lengthening your legs as you stand or lunge in postures such as Warrior 1, Warrior 2, and Mountain allows blood in your body to more easily circulate downward. Other grounding yoga poses involve drawing your pelvis or center of gravity toward the earth as if you're rooting yourself or landing into the posture. One example of this technique is Pigeon, described below. Here's a sequence to stimulate grounding energy. Remember to begin your session by doing the Strength Sun Salutation two times, and to end your practice with Relaxation, Grounding Breath, and then the Three-Seal Breathing technique.

GROUNDING SEQUENCE SUMMARY —

1. Mountain

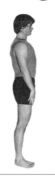

2. Extended Mountain

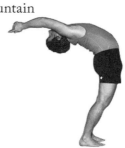

3. Standing Forward Bend

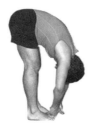

4. Gazing Halfway Up

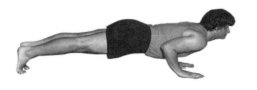

5. Long Staff

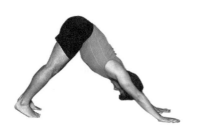

6. Upward Dog

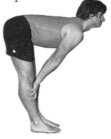

7. Downward Dog

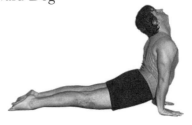

8. One-Legged Downward Dog (right leg up)

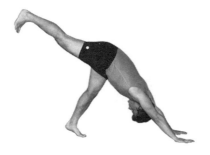

9. Pigeon (right knee forward)

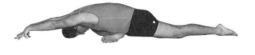

10. One-Legged Downward Dog (left leg up)

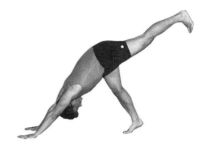

11. Pigeon (left knee forward)

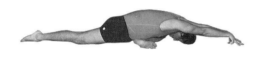

12. Downward Dog

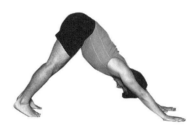

13. Gazing Halfway Up

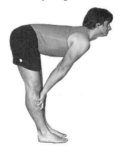

14. Standing Forward Bend

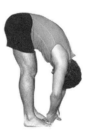

15. Extended Mountain

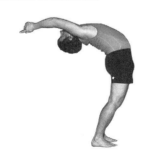

16. Mountain ✦

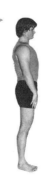

STRENGTH SUN SALUTATION

Do 2 repetitions of the Strength Sun Salutation to warm up.

— GROUNDING SEQUENCE —

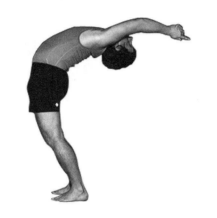

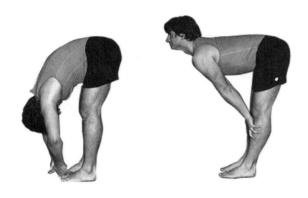

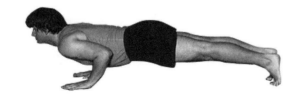

1. Begin in **Mountain**.

2. **Extended Mountain:** As you inhale, reach your arms up over your head, shoulder-distance apart, and extend back into a gentle arch.

3. **Standing Forward Bend:** As you exhale, hinge forward from your hips and place your hands on your shins, ankles, or feet, or on the floor, as you are able. Drop your head and soften the back of your neck.

4. **Gazing Halfway Up:** Inhale and gaze halfway up directly in front of you, elongating your spine and working toward a slight arch if you're able.

5. **Long Staff:** Exhale and, with your hands on the ground shoulder-width apart, step your feet behind you hip-distance apart, so that your body is in one straight line; think of it as a horizontal version of **Mountain**, with your knees, hips, and shoulders aligned. Bend your elbows, keeping them by your sides, to lower your body a few inches above the ground. Gaze forward and keep your thigh muscles engaged and your belly in.

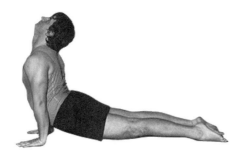

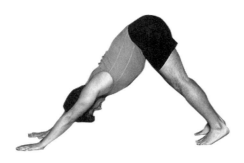

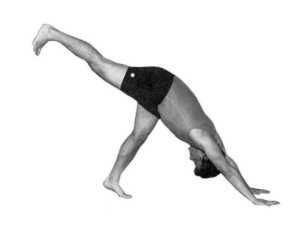

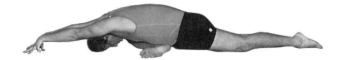

6. **Upward Dog:** As you inhale, lift and press your chest forward and up, dropping your shoulder blades to keep your shoulders back and down and keeping the tops of your toes and feet on the floor.

7. **Downward Dog:** Exhale, curl your toes under, and lift your sit bones up toward the ceiling, straightening your legs. Keep your back long and gaze through your extended legs.

8. **One-Legged Downward Dog (right leg up):** Transfer your weight to your left foot and lift your right leg back and up into the air, keeping it extended, and keeping your left heel grounded if possible. Hold for 3 breaths, then return your right foot to the floor and come to an all fours position.

9. **Pigeon (right knee forward):** Bring your right knee forward just inside your right hand, angling your lower leg toward the left so you rest on the outside of your right shin. Point your hips squarely toward the floor as you extend your left leg behind you, with the top of the foot and knee touching the floor. Inhale and lift your chest, keeping your arms elongated and your hands on the floor. Exhale and hinge forward, bringing your forehead to the floor with your arms stretched out beyond your head and keeping both hip bones pointing down to the floor. Hold for 5 to 12 breaths. Inhale and walk your hands toward your knees, lifting your chest, then return to an all-fours position.

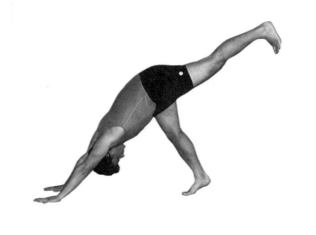

10. **One-Legged Downward Dog (left leg up):** Exhale, curl your toes under, and lift your sit bones up toward the ceiling into **Downward Dog,** straightening your legs, then transfer your weight to your right foot and lift your left leg back and up into the air, keeping it extended, and keeping your right heel grounded if possible. Hold for 3 breaths, then return your left foot to the floor and come to an all-fours position.

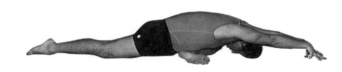

11. **Pigeon (left knee forward):** Bring your left knee forward just inside your left hand, angling your lower leg toward the left so you rest on the outside of your left shin. Point your hips squarely toward the floor as you extend your right leg behind you, with the top of the foot and knee touching the floor. Inhale and lift your chest, keeping your arms elongated and your hands on the floor. Exhale and hinge forward, bringing your forehead to the floor with your arms stretched out beyond your head and keeping both hip bones pointing down to the floor. Hold for 5 to 12 breaths.

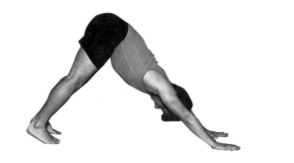

12. **Downward Dog:** Inhale and walk your hands toward your knees, lifting your chest, then return to an all-fours position. Exhale, curl your toes under, and lift your sit bones up toward the ceiling, straightening your legs. Keep your back long and gaze through your extended legs.

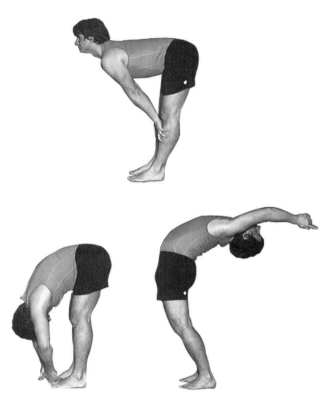

13. **Gazing Halfway Up:** Inhale and step your feet up to a position between your hands, with knees bent if necessary. Straighten your legs, keeping your hands on the floor or resting them on your ankles or shins. Gaze halfway up directly in front of you, elongating and gently arching your spine.

14. **Standing Forward Bend:** Exhale, relax your neck and back, and bring your chest and belly button toward your legs.

15. **Extended Mountain:** Inhale and return to an upright position, keeping your spine long and sweeping your arms up over your head, shoulder-distance apart. Extend back into a gentle arch.

16. **Mountain:** Exhale and return to Mountain, with your arms by your sides, for 1 breath.

17. Repeat the entire sequence 4 more times. ✦

— RELAXATION POSE —

1. Lie on your back with your legs straight and your arms by your sides.

2. Bring your legs out until your feet are a little farther than hip-width apart.

3. Take your arms out until they're at about a 30-degree angle from your sides, palms facing up. You may also rest your hands on your belly if you prefer.

4. Tuck your chin slightly into your chest while lengthening through the back of your head and neck.

5. Remain in this position for at least 5 minutes, letting your body relax as much as possible. Breathe naturally and make sure you always exhale slowly. ◆

— GROUNDING BREATH —

The exhalation phase of breath is associated with calming or grounding. Breathing techniques that emphasize exhaling or a pause at the end of exhalation, such as this one, stimulate grounded energy.

1. Sit comfortably with your spine long.

2. Inhale naturally.

3. As you exhale, make your breath longer and slower.

4. At the end of your exhalation, hold your breath while applying a chin seal for 2 to 3 seconds, tucking your chin 20 degrees down toward your throat. Release the chin seal.

5. Steps 2 through 4 comprise 1 round. Repeat for a total of 8 to 12 rounds. ◆

— THREE-SEAL BREATHING —

1. Sit in a comfortable cross-legged position on the floor with your spine long or sit in a chair with the back of the chair supporting your back.

2. Close your eyes. Breathe in and out through your nose.

3. As you inhale, contract your perineum by squeezing your anal sphincter to engage the root seal.

4. At the end of your inhale, draw your chin down 20 degrees and retract your head slightly so your ears align over your shoulders to engage the chin seal.

5. As you exhale, maintain both the root seal and the chin seal.

6. At the end of your exhalation, rapidly draw your belly in and up to engage the navel seal.

7. Inhale and release all three seals. Exhale naturally. ◆

ENERGY FLOW: CORE

Visualize core energy as a circular flow around your waist, where energy that's housed in your abdomen moves from the external to the internal. The natural element associated with core energy is fire. Healthy core energy helps your body burn away toxins. The theory behind this energy system is that you fan digestive fires with your exhalation while activating your core by drawing your belly in.

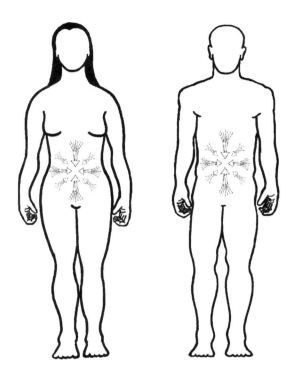

Core energy draws inward, creating a gateway to deeper dimensions of your being. This outward-to-inward motion leads to the experience of feeling centered—a state that encourages optimal alignment, both mentally and physically. For example, the simple act of drawing your attention inward can realign your body as you focus on what feels right and what needs to be tweaked.

On a physical level, better alignment will make your asana practice more efficient and enjoyable because you'll be better able to stretch and strengthen your muscles without strain. In terms of energetics, being well-aligned helps energy flow more easily through your body. Think of someone who's slumped forward with a rounded back and shoulders. Would you imagine that person has strong internal energy? Probably not. Now visualize someone who stands upright with shoulders back and head held high. That type of posture naturally allows energy to increase and flow more efficiently. Good alignment during asana practice produces the same effect.

CORE SEQUENCE

Poses that support activation of the core muscles at the end of exhalation stimulate core energy. These poses include forward bends, such as Standing Forward Bend. Postures that require you to balance are also good for engaging the core. Here's a sequence to stimulate core energy. Remember to begin your session by doing the Strength Sun Salutation two times, and to end your practice with Relaxation, Core Breath, and then the Three-Seal Breathing technique.

CORE SEQUENCE SUMMARY (*Perform 5 times.*) —

1. Mountain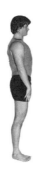

2. Extended Mountain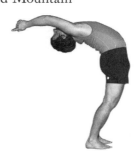

3. Standing Forward Bend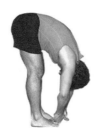

4. Gazing Halfway Up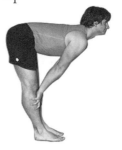

5. Long Staff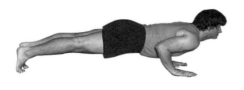

6. Upward Dog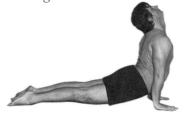

7. Downward Dog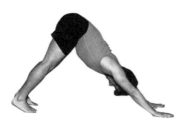

8. Beginner Accomplished Pose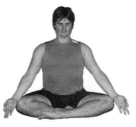

9. Seated Hand to Big Toe

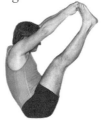

10. Seated Legs Up and Apart

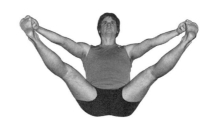

11. Repeat 9 and 10 three more times

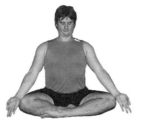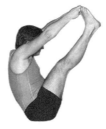

12. Beginner Accomplished Pose

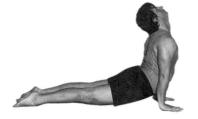

13. Long Staff

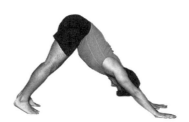

14. Upward Dog

15. Downward Dog

16. Gazing Halfway Up

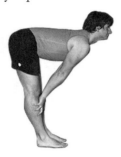

17. Standing Forward Bend

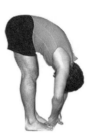

18. Extended Mountain

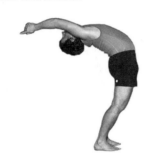

19. Mountain ◆

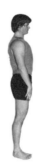

After 5 repetitions, end with this sequence:

1. Relaxation Pose
2. Core Breath
3. Three-Seal Breathing

Strength Sun Salutation

Do 2 repetitions of the Strength Sun Salutation to warm up.

— Core Sequence —

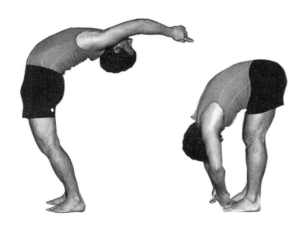

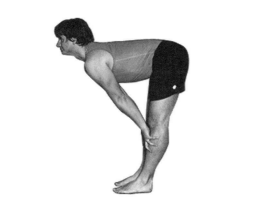

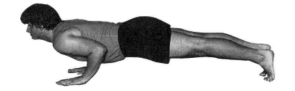

1. Begin in **Mountain**.

2. **Extended Mountain:** As you inhale, reach your arms up over your head, shoulder-distance apart, and extend back into a gentle arch.

3. **Standing Forward Bend:** As you exhale, hinge forward from your hips and place your hands on your shins, ankles, or feet, or on the floor, as you are able. Drop your head and soften the back of your neck.

4. **Gazing Halfway Up:** Inhale and gaze halfway up directly in front of you, elongating your spine and working toward a slight arch if you're able.

5. **Long Staff:** Exhale and, with your hands on the ground shoulder-width apart, step your feet behind you hip-distance apart, so that your body is in one straight line; think of it as a horizontal version of **Mountain**, with your knees, hips, and shoulders aligned. Bend your elbows, keeping them by your sides, to lower your body a few inches above the ground. Gaze forward and keep your thigh muscles engaged and your belly in.

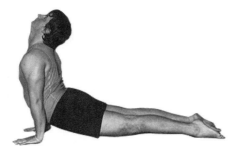

6. **Upward Dog:** As you inhale, lift and press your chest forward and up, dropping your shoulder blades to keep your shoulders back and down and keeping the tops of your toes and feet on the floor.

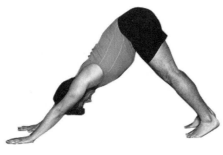

7. **Downward Dog:** Exhale, curl your toes under, and lift your sit bones up toward the ceiling, straightening your legs. Keep your back long and gaze through your extended legs.

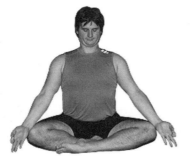

8. **Beginner Accomplished Pose:** Jump or walk your feet through your hands and come into **Beginner Accomplished Pose,** sitting cross-legged with your right heel slightly to the left of the midline of your body and your left heel slightly to the right of the midline of your body. Hold your spine upright and long and press your thighs toward the floor. Hold for 1 breath.

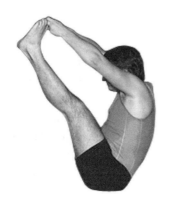

9. **Seated Hand to Big Toe:** Extend your legs in front of you, then bend your legs slightly and use your first two fingers to grab your big toes. Inhale, lean back slightly off your sit bones, and extend your legs toward the ceiling while rounding your back slightly and keeping your legs together. Hold for 5 to 12 breaths.

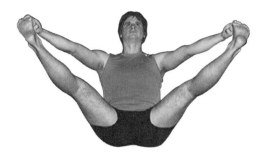

10. **Seated Legs Up and Apart:** Inhale again and open your legs out to the sides, bringing your spine into a slight arch as you do so. Bend your knees a bit if you need to. Hold for 5 to 12 breaths.

11. Repeat steps 9 and 10 three more times, holding for only 1 breath each time.

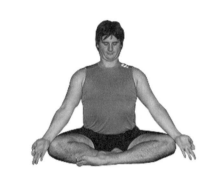

12. **Beginner Accomplished Pose** Keeping your fingers interlaced around your big toes, bend your legs and bring them back down into **Beginner Accomplished Pose**. Rest your hands on your thighs and hold for 3 to 5 breaths.

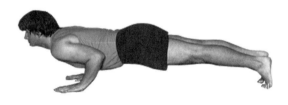

13. **Long Staff:** Exhale, put your palms on the floor in front of you, shoulder-distance apart, and jump or step your feet back into **Long Staff**, with your body in one straight line. Bend your elbows to lower your body a few inches above the ground and gaze forward, keeping your thigh muscles engaged and your belly in.

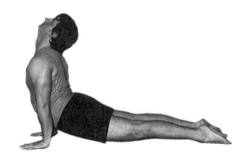

14. **Upward Dog:** As you inhale, lift and press your chest forward and up, dropping your shoulder blades to keep your shoulders back and down and keeping the tops of your toes and feet on the floor.

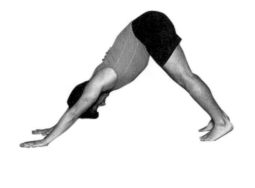

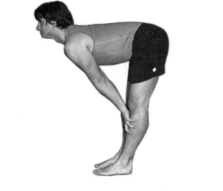

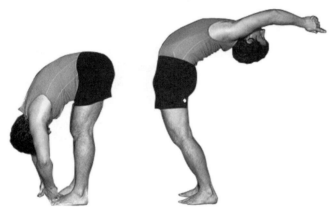

15. **Downward Dog:** Exhale, curl your toes under, and lift your sit bones up toward the ceiling, straightening your legs. Keep your back long and gaze through your extended legs.

16. **Gazing Halfway Up:** Inhale and step your feet up to a position between your hands, with knees bent if necessary. Straighten your legs, keeping your hands on the floor or resting them on your ankles or shins. Gaze halfway up directly in front of you, elongating and gently arching your spine.

17. **Standing Forward Bend:** Exhale, relax your neck and back, and bring your chest and belly button toward your legs.

18. **Extended Mountain:** Inhale and return to an upright position, keeping your spine long and sweeping your arms up over your head, shoulder-distance apart. Extend back into a gentle arch.

19. **Mountain:** Exhale and return to Mountain, with your arms by your sides, for 1 breath.

20. Repeat the entire sequence 4 more times. ✦

— RELAXATION POSE —

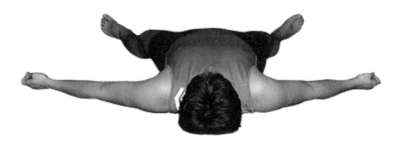

1. Lie on your back with your legs straight and your arms by your sides.

2. Bring your legs out until your feet are a little farther than hip-width apart.

3. Take your arms out until they're at about a 30-degree angle from your sides, palms facing up. You may also rest your hands on your belly if you prefer.

4. Tuck your chin slightly into your chest while lengthening through the back of your head and neck.

5. Remain in this position for at least 5 minutes, letting your body relax as much as possible. Breathe naturally and make sure you always exhale slowly. ◆

— CORE BREATH —

Inhaling deeply tends to invigorate you, while exhaling has a more calming effect. Core energy is associated with breathing exercises that accentuate exhaling to create a sense of serenity.

1. Sit comfortably with your spine long. Place your right palm on your navel.

2. Inhale naturally.

3. As you exhale, draw your belly in and up as if scooping under your rib cage.

4. On your next inhale, make sure the breath is smooth and long.

5. Steps 3 and 4 comprise 1 round. Repeat for a total of 12 rounds.

6. Relax and breathe naturally for 1 minute, then do 2 more cycles of 12 rounds each. ◆

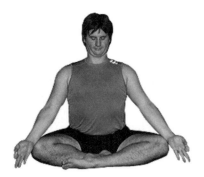

— THREE-SEAL BREATHING —

1. Sit in a comfortable cross-legged position on the floor with your spine long or sit in a chair with the back of the chair supporting your back.

2. Close your eyes. Breathe in and out through your nose.

3. As you inhale, contract your perineum by squeezing your anal sphincter to engage the root seal.

4. At the end of your inhale, draw your chin down 20 degrees and retract your head slightly so your ears align over your shoulders to engage the chin seal.

5. As you exhale, maintain both the root seal and the chin seal.

6. At the end of your exhalation, rapidly draw your belly in and up to engage the navel seal.

7. Inhale and release all three seals. Exhale naturally. ◆

ENERGY FLOW: CLARITY

The energy flow that represents clarity is concentrated in the throat and up to the crown of the head, flowing upward in a one-directional path. Its natural element is ether, which has an atmospheric quality of space and expansiveness—words I would also use to describe mental clarity. Basically, it's the opposite of a closed, cluttered mind.

If your clarity current is blocked, you might feel a sense of confusion, or as though your head is full of junk. It's hard to feel positive when your head is in that state. Healthy, clearheaded energy, on the other hand, helps you adopt a positive attitude, where you can choose thoughts that make you feel good. This power of choice broadens the imagination. It's also a prevailing theme in yogic philosophy because it helps channel divine inspiration, or Atman. I'll expand on the concept of choosing positive thinking in the next chapter, which deals with the meditation kosha.

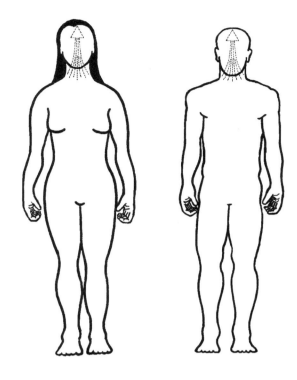

In addition to clearheadedness, this energy flow is manifested in speech and singing. You'll see why these aspects are linked when you try the breathing exercise for clarity. It encourages you to use your voice—chanting "om"—in addition to your breath for energy stimulation.

CLARITY SEQUENCE

Postures that stimulate clarity are those that direct the crown of your head toward the earth, creating more awareness in that area of your body. Any pose that helps move blood toward and into the head and neck area will be helpful, such as the Shoulder Stand, Headstand, and Standing Forward Bend. Here's a sequence to stimulate clarity. Remember to begin your session by doing the Strength Sun Salutation two times, and to end your practice with Relaxation, Clarity Breath, and then the Three-Seal Breathing technique.

CLARITY SEQUENCE SUMMARY *(Perform 5 times.)* —

1. Mountain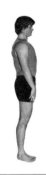

2. Extended Mountain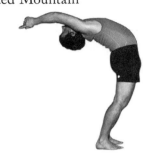

3. Standing Forward Bend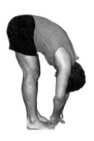

4. Gazing Halfway Up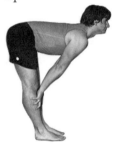

5. Long Staff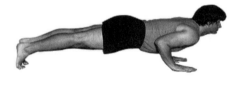

6. Upward Dog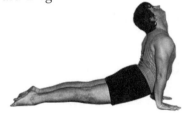

7. Downward Dog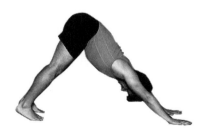

8. Headstand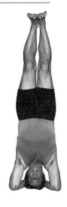

9. Child's Pose

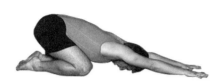

12. Downward Dog

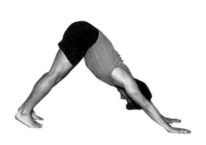

13. Gazing Halfway Up

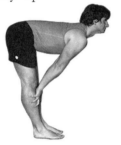

14. Standing Forward Bend

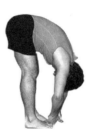

15. Extended Mountain

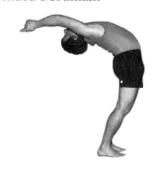

16. Mountain ◆

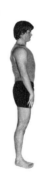

After 5 repetitions, end with this sequence:

1. Relaxation Pose

2. Clarity Breath

3. Three-Seal Breathing

STRENGTH SUN SALUTATION

Do 2 repetitions of the Strength Sun Salutation to warm up.

— CLARITY SEQUENCE —

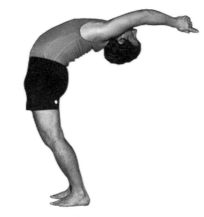
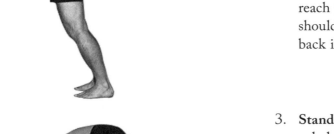

1. Begin in **Mountain**.

2. **Extended Mountain:** As you inhale, reach your arms up over your head, shoulder-distance apart, and extend back into a gentle arch.

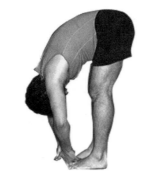

3. **Standing Forward Bend:** As you exhale, hinge forward from your hips and place your hands on your shins, ankles, or feet, or on the floor, as you are able. Drop your head and soften the back of your neck.

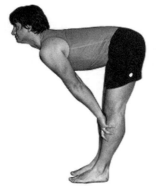

4. **Gazing Halfway Up:** Inhale and gaze halfway up directly in front of you, elongating your spine and working toward a slight arch if you're able.

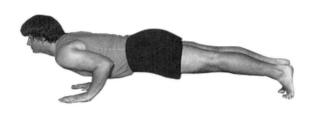

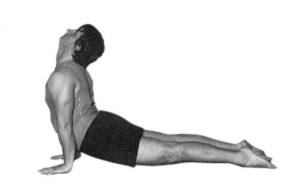

5. **Long Staff:** Exhale and, with your hands on the ground shoulder-width apart, step your feet behind you hip-distance apart, so that your body is in one straight line; think of it as a horizontal version of **Mountain**, with your knees, hips, and shoulders aligned. Bend your elbows, keeping them by your sides, to lower your body a few inches above the ground. Gaze forward and keep your thigh muscles engaged and your belly in.

6. **Upward Dog:** As you inhale, lift and press your chest forward and up, dropping your shoulder blades to keep your shoulders back and down and keeping the tops of your toes and feet on the floor.

7. **Downward Dog:** Exhale, curl your toes under, and lift your sit bones up toward the ceiling, straightening your legs. Keep your back long and gaze through your extended legs.

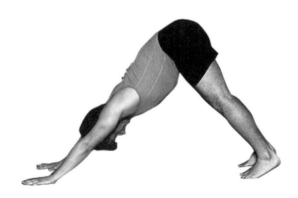

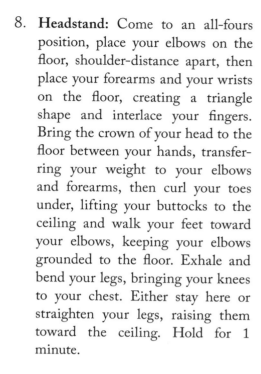
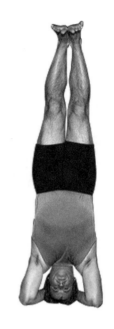

8. **Headstand:** Come to an all-fours position, place your elbows on the floor, shoulder-distance apart, then place your forearms and your wrists on the floor, creating a triangle shape and interlace your fingers. Bring the crown of your head to the floor between your hands, transferring your weight to your elbows and forearms, then curl your toes under, lifting your buttocks to the ceiling and walk your feet toward your elbows, keeping your elbows grounded to the floor. Exhale and bend your legs, bringing your knees to your chest. Either stay here or straighten your legs, raising them toward the ceiling. Hold for 1 minute.

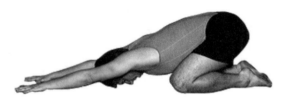

9. **Child's Pose:** Exhale and lower one leg at a time to the floor. Bring your buttocks to your heels and rest your forehead on the floor in **Child's Pose**, with your arms by your sides or stretched over your head. Hold for 3 to 5 breaths.

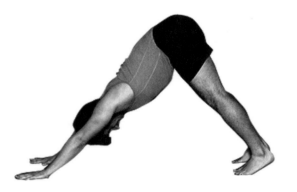

10. **Downward Dog:** Come up into an all-fours position, then exhale, curl your toes under, and lift your sit bones up toward the ceiling, straightening your legs. Keep your back long and gaze through your extended legs.

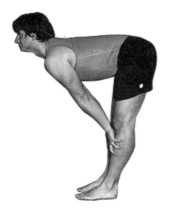

11. **Gazing Halfway Up:** Inhale and step your feet up to a position between your hands, with knees bent if necessary. Straighten your legs, keeping your hands on the floor or resting them on your ankles or shins. Gaze halfway up directly in front of you, elongating and gently arching your spine.

12. **Standing Forward Bend:** Exhale, relax your neck and back, and bring your chest and belly button toward your legs.

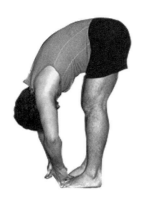

13. **Extended Mountain:** Inhale and return to an upright position, keeping your spine long and sweeping your arms up over your head, shoulder-distance apart. Extend back into a gentle arch.

14. **Mountain:** Exhale and return to **Mountain,** with your arms by your sides, for 1 breath.

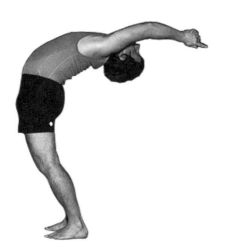

15. Repeat the entire sequence 4 more times. ◆

— RELAXATION POSE —

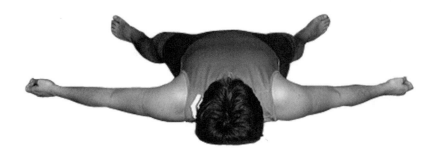

1. Lie on your back with your legs straight and your arms by your sides.

2. Bring your legs out until your feet are a little farther than hip-width apart.

3. Take your arms out until they're at about a 30-degree angle from your sides, palms facing up. You may also rest your hands on your belly if you prefer.

4. Tuck your chin slightly into your chest while lengthening through the back of your head and neck.

5. Remain in this position for at least 5 minutes, letting your body relax as much as possible. Breathe naturally and make sure you always exhale slowly. ✦

— CLARITY BREATH —

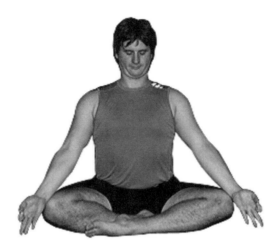

For this breathing exercise, you'll practice a continuous "om," where you say—almost sing, really—"om" for as long as your exhalation will allow. Since exhalation has a calming effect, this exercise is especially good for quelling anxiety because adding sound helps draw out the exhalation. The word "om" sounds like "aum." Let the "aaaaaaaa" and "uuuuuuu" be the longest part of the word. The "m" sound should last for only a couple of seconds.

1. Sit comfortably with your spine long.

2. Inhale naturally. Exhale and say "om" at the same time. Keep the sound going for as long as you comfortably can.

3. Inhale again, slowly and quietly.

4. Repeat for 3 to 10 minutes. ◆

— THREE-SEAL BREATHING —

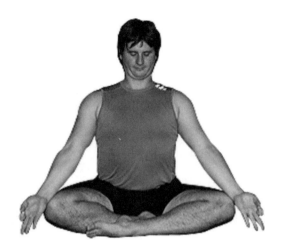

1. Sit in a comfortable cross-legged position on the floor with your spine long or sit in a chair with the back of the chair supporting your back.

2. Close your eyes. Breathe in and out through your nose.

3. As you inhale, contract your perineum by squeezing your anal sphincter to engage the root seal.

4. At the end of your inhale, draw your chin down 20 degrees and retract your head slightly so your ears align over your shoulders to engage the chin seal.

5. As you exhale, maintain both the root seal and the chin seal.

6. At the end of your exhalation, rapidly draw your belly in and up to engage the navel seal.

7. Inhale and release all three seals. Exhale naturally. ◆

Energy Flow: Vitality

The energy current for vitality runs upward, from your belly button to your heart. Its corresponding natural element is air. On a physiological level, when you breathe deeply, you nourish your body's cells with oxygen. You literally breathe in energy. If you're breathing to your full potential with deep, expansive breaths, your vitality increases. If, on the other hand, your breathing is shallow, your vitality is lost or diminished.

The fact that this vital energy flow originates from your body's powerful center, the navel, is especially significant. You've probably noticed from your physical yoga practice that activating your core by drawing your belly in helps you remain strong and stable within a pose. Similarly, you can draw much of your energetic power from your navel.

From the navel, vital energy rises to the heart—a symbol of life, but also of love and compassion for self and others. Between the navel and the heart

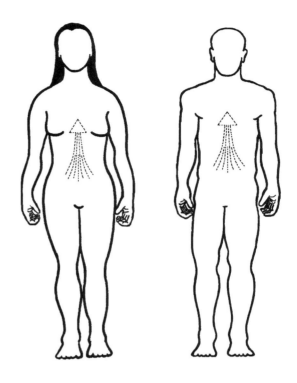

lies the solar plexus, which is thought to be the seat or foundation of willpower. Willpower confers the ability to change aspects of yourself with intention and deliberateness. It deepens your faith and resolve. With that in mind, consider how stirring up your vital energy—ensuring it doesn't sit stagnant—opens your heart to change and personal enlightenment. Simply put, for change to occur, you must invite change. Strong vital energy is one step toward that readiness.

VITALITY SEQUENCE

To stimulate vital energy, follow the sequence presented below. It contains the Full Wheel, a backbend that opens and frees vital energy in the body. Extending your spine in a backbend lets you expand your lungs so you inhale more deeply. It also expands your chest and opens your heart center, an important theme for this energy flow. Remember to begin your session by doing the Strength Sun Salutation two times, and to end your practice with Relaxation, Vitality Breath, and then the Three-Seal Breathing technique.

VITALITY SEQUENCE SUMMARY (*Perform 5 times.*) ——

1. Mountain
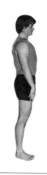

2. Extended Mountain
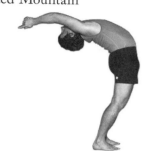

3. Standing Forward Bend
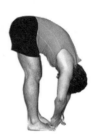

4. Gazing Halfway Up
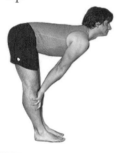

5. Long Staff
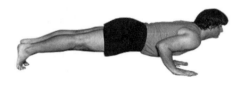

6. Upward Dog
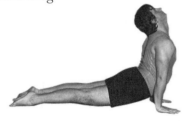

7. Downward Dog
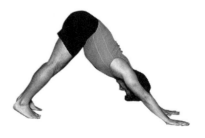

8. Beginner Accomplished Pose
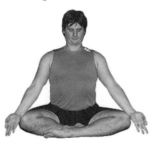

9. Full Wheel

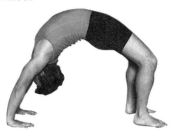

10. Knees to Chest

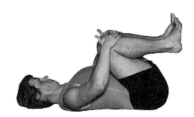

11. Beginner Accomplished Pose

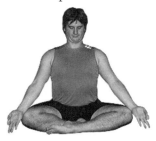

12. Downward Dog

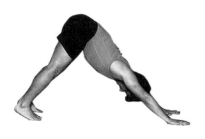

13. Gazing Halfway Up

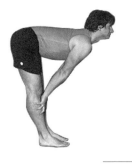

14. Standing Forward Bend

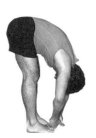

15. Extended Mountain

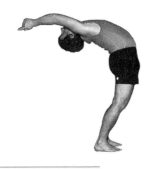

16. Mountain ◆

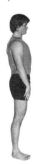

After 5 repetitions, end with this sequence:

1. Relaxation Pose

2. Vitality Breath

3. Three-Seal Breathing

STRENGTH SUN SALUTATION

Do 2 repetitions of the Strength Sun Salutation to warm up.

— VITALITY SEQUENCE —

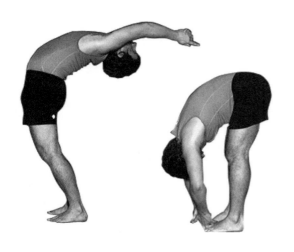

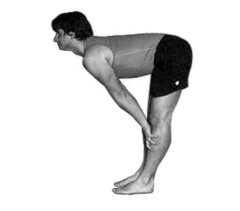

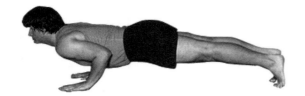

1. Begin in **Mountain**.

2. **Extended Mountain:** As you inhale, reach your arms up over your head, shoulder-distance apart, and extend back into a gentle arch.

3. **Standing Forward Bend:** As you exhale, hinge forward from your hips and place your hands on your shins, ankles, or feet, or on the floor, as you are able. Drop your head and soften the back of your neck.

4. **Gazing Halfway Up:** Inhale and gaze halfway up directly in front of you, elongating your spine and working toward a slight arch if you're able.

5. **Long Staff:** Exhale and, with your hands on the ground shoulder-width apart, step your feet behind you hip-distance apart, so that your body is in one straight line; think of it as a horizontal version of **Mountain**, with your knees, hips, and shoulders aligned. Bend your elbows, keeping them by your sides, to lower your body a few inches above the ground. Gaze forward and keep your thigh muscles engaged and your belly in.

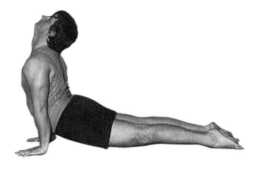

6. **Upward Dog:** As you inhale, lift and press your chest forward and up, dropping your shoulder blades to keep your shoulders back and down and keeping the tops of your toes and feet on the floor.

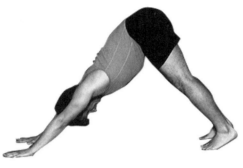

7. **Downward Dog:** Exhale, curl your toes under, and lift your sit bones up toward the ceiling, straightening your legs. Keep your back long and gaze through your extended legs.

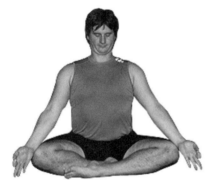

8. **Beginner Accomplished Pose:** Jump or walk your feet through your hands and come into Beginner Accomplished Pose, sitting cross-legged with your right heel slightly to the left of the midline of your body and your left heel slightly to the right of the midline of your body. Hold your spine upright and long and press your thighs toward the floor. Hold for 1 breath.

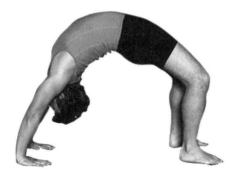

9. **Full Wheel:** Lie on your back with your legs bent, feet on the floor with your heels as close to your buttocks as possible. Place your hands under your shoulders with your palms down and fingers pointing toward your feet. Inhale and use your arms and legs to arch your back off the floor, with the crown of your head touching the floor. Your elbows should be bent and about shoulder-distance apart, rather than splaying out. Exhale, then inhale and straighten your arms, lifting your head off the floor and pressing through your feet as you arch your back. Hold for 5 to 12 breaths.

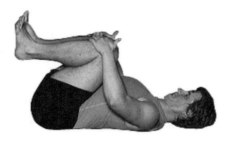

10. **Knees to Chest:** Bend your elbows and tuck your chin in as you lower your head to the floor, then gradually bring your upper back, then mid back, then lower back to the floor. Hug your knees to your chest, keeping your sacrum against the floor and your chin tucked slightly in. Hold for 3 to 5 breaths.

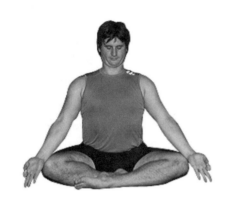

11. **Beginner Accomplished Pose:** Grab your knees and roll up to a seated position, coming back into **Beginner Accomplished Pose.** Hold for 1 breath.

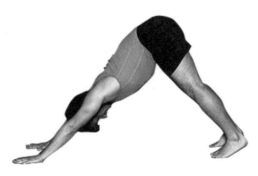

12. **Downward Dog:** Get on your hands and knees, then exhale, curl your toes under, and lift your sit bones up toward the ceiling, straightening your legs. Keep your back long and gaze through your extended legs.

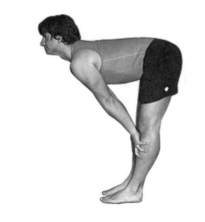

13. **Gazing Halfway Up:** Inhale and step your feet up to a position between your hands, with knees bent if necessary. Straighten your legs, keeping your hands on the floor or resting them on your ankles or shins. Gaze halfway up directly in front of you, elongating and gently arching your spine.

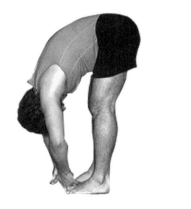

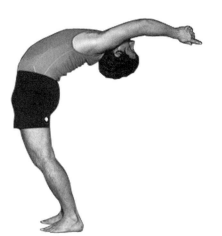

14. **Standing Forward Bend:** Exhale, relax your neck and back, and bring your chest and belly button toward your legs.

15. **Extended Mountain:** Inhale and return to an upright position, keeping your spine long and sweeping your arms up over your head, shoulder-distance apart. Extend back into a gentle arch.

16. **Mountain:** Exhale and return to Mountain, with your arms by your sides, for 1 breath.

17. Repeat the entire sequence 4 more times. ◆

— RELAXATION POSE —

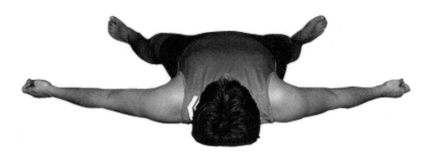

1. Lie on your back with your legs straight and your arms by your sides.

2. Bring your legs out until your feet are a little farther than hip-width apart.

3. Take your arms out until they're at about a 30-degree angle from your sides, palms facing up. You may also rest your hands on your belly if you prefer.

4. Tuck your chin slightly into your chest while lengthening through the back of your head and neck.

5. Remain in this position for at least 5 minutes, letting your body relax as much as possible. Breathe naturally and make sure you always exhale slowly. ◆

— VITALITY BREATH —

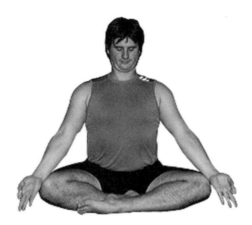

Since the natural element for vitality is air, the breathing exercise for this energy system focuses on allowing a full expansion of both your diaphragm and your lungs with each inhalation. As you'll see below, using your hands as a guide helps you feel your lungs fill with vital air.

1. Sit comfortably with your spine long.

2. Create an L shape with each hand, fingers together and thumbs extended. Place your palms on your breastbone with your thumbs in your underarms and your middle fingertips touching.

3. As you inhale, expand your rib cage and chest so your right and left fingertips move away from each other, creating a slight gap between your fingertips.

4. At the top of the inhale, hold your breath for 2 to 3 seconds maximum.

5. Exhale naturally, in a smooth, controlled way, rather than releasing air too fast or gasping for the next breath.

6. Steps 3 and 4 comprise 1 round. Repeat for a maximum of 8 rounds. It isn't a good idea to do more, as you could overstimulate your nervous system. ✦

— THREE-SEAL BREATHING —

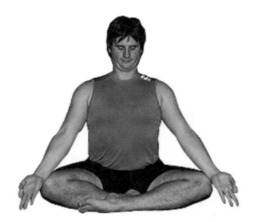

1. Sit in a comfortable cross-legged position on the floor with your spine long or sit in a chair with the back of the chair supporting your back.

2. Close your eyes. Breathe in and out through your nose.

3. As you inhale, contract your perineum by squeezing your anal sphincter to engage the root seal.

4. At the end of your inhale, draw your chin down 20 degrees and retract your head slightly so your ears align over your shoulders to engage the chin seal.

5. As you exhale, maintain both the root seal and the chin seal.

6. At the end of your exhalation, rapidly draw your belly in and up to engage the navel seal.

7. Inhale and release all three seals. Exhale naturally. ✦

ENERGY FLOW: WHOLENESS

Wholeness energy aids in proper circulation and skin tone. It stems from the navel, extending to your arms and hands, your legs and feet, and the top of your head. Imagine this energy flow coursing throughout your entire body, through every space and every blood vessel. Essentially, this energy is what helps you feel whole.

The previous four energy systems involve drawing your attention to specific sites in your body. The purpose of wholeness is to sense energy as a far-reaching, interconnected force. Since water is the natural element associated with wholeness, I like to think of it as being similar to an ocean—deep, vast, and wide open. You may also think of wholeness as the absence of a feeling of separation. When you're whole, you're connected to something greater than your ego self: Atman.

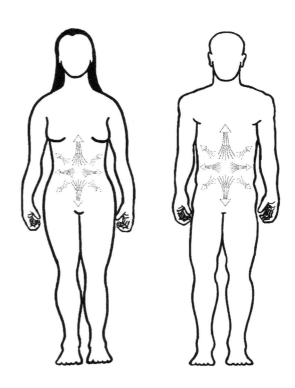

WHOLENESS SEQUENCE

The Goddess posture is known for stimulating wholeness because of the way it opens the body. This pose accentuates both grounding and stability as well as reaching and lengthening toward the heavens for an awareness of your entire physical being. The effect is a body that's open, both physically and in terms of energetics. Here's a sequence to stimulate wholeness. Remember to begin your session by doing the Strength Sun Salutation two times, and to end your practice with Relaxation, Wholeness Breath, and then the Three-Seal Breathing technique.

WHOLENESS SEQUENCE SUMMARY (*Perform 5 times.*) —

1. Mountain

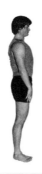

2. Extended Mountain

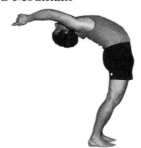

3. Standing Forward Bend

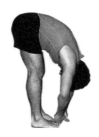

4. Gazing Halfway Up

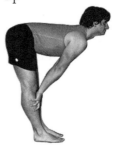

5. Long Staff

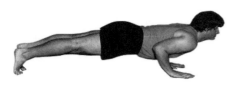

6. Upward Dog

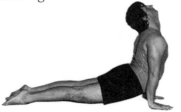

7. Downward Dog

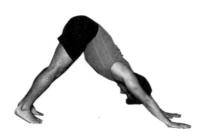

8. Gazing Halfway Up

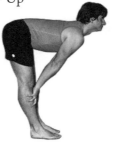

9. Standing Forward Bend

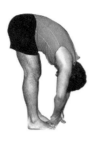

10. Extended Mountain

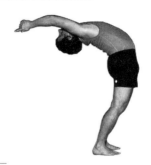

11. Mountain

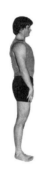

12. Goddess

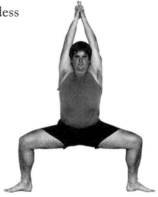

13. Mountain ◆

After 5 repetitions, end with this sequence:

1. Relaxation Pose

2. Wholeness Breath

3. Three-Seal Breathing

Strength Sun Salutation

Do 2 repetitions of the Strength Sun Salutation to warm up.

— Wholeness Sequence —

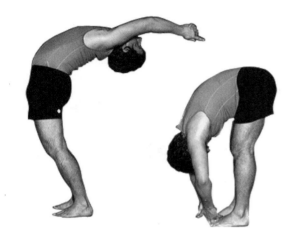

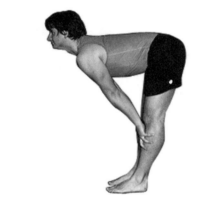

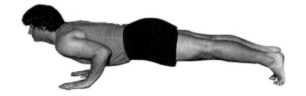

1. Begin in **Mountain**.

2. **Extended Mountain:** As you inhale, reach your arms up over your head, shoulder-distance apart, and extend back into a gentle arch.

3. **Standing Forward Bend:** As you exhale, hinge forward from your hips and place your hands on your shins, ankles, or feet, or on the floor, as you are able. Drop your head and soften the back of your neck.

4. **Gazing Halfway Up:** Inhale and gaze halfway up directly in front of you, elongating your spine and working toward a slight arch if you're able.

5. **Long Staff:** Exhale and, with your hands on the ground shoulder-width apart, step your feet back behind you hip-distance apart, so that your body is in one straight line; think of it as a horizontal version of **Mountain**, with your knees, hips, and shoulders aligned. Bend your elbows, keeping them by your sides, to lower your body a few inches above the ground. Gaze forward and keep your thigh muscles engaged and your belly in.

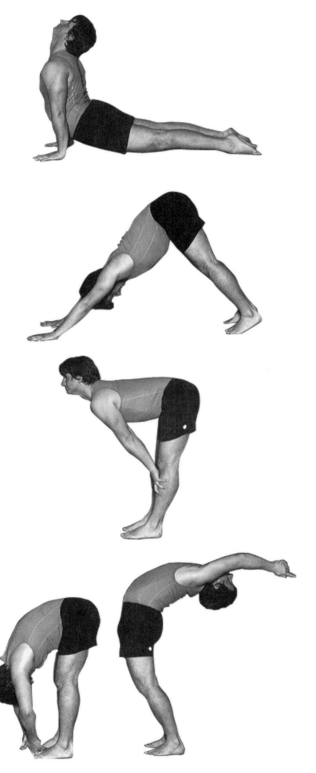

6. **Upward Dog:** As you inhale, lift and press your chest forward and up, dropping your shoulder blades to keep your shoulders back and down and keeping the tops of your toes and feet on the floor.

7. **Downward Dog:** Exhale, curl your toes under, and lift your sit bones up toward the ceiling, straightening your legs. Keep your back long and gaze through your extended legs.

8. **Gazing Halfway Up:** Inhale and step your feet up to a position between your hands, with knees bent if necessary. Straighten your legs, keeping your hands on the floor or resting them on your ankles or shins. Gaze halfway up directly in front of you, elongating and gently arching your spine.

9. **Standing Forward Bend:** Exhale, relax your neck and back, and bring your chest and belly button toward your legs.

10. **Extended Mountain:** Inhale and return to an upright position, keeping your spine long and sweeping your arms up over your head, shoulder-distance apart. Extend back into a gentle arch.

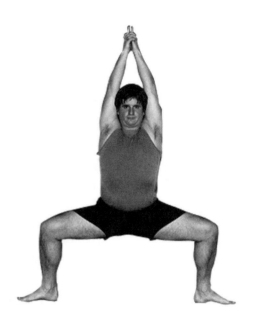

11. **Mountain:** Exhale and return to **Mountain**, with your arms by your sides.

12. **Goddess:** Turn 90 degrees to the right, to face the long side of the mat. Inhale, step your right foot out about 3 feet to the side, then turn your feet out so your toes point toward the ends of the mat. Exhale and bend your knees to about 90 degrees, keeping your knees aligned over your ankles. Reach your arms over your head, placing your palms together, and pressing up through your index fingers. Hold for 5 to 12 breaths, deepening into the pose each time you exhale. Straighten your legs and bring your arms to your sides, then step your right foot back beside your left foot.

13. **Mountain:** Turn to face the front of the mat in **Mountain** with your arms by your sides. Rest and recenter in **Mountain** for 3 breaths.

14. Repeat the entire sequence 4 more times. ◆

— Relaxation Pose —

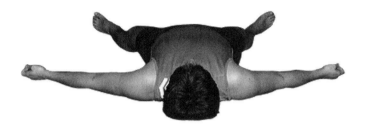

1. Lie on your back with your legs straight and your arms by your sides.

2. Bring your legs out until your feet are a little farther than hip-width apart.

3. Take your arms out until they're at about a 30-degree angle from your sides, palms facing up. You may also rest your hands on your belly if you prefer.

4. Tuck your chin slightly into your chest while lengthening through the back of your head and neck.

5. Remain in this position for at least 5 minutes, letting your body relax as much as possible. Breathe naturally and make sure you always exhale slowly. ◆

— Wholeness Breath —

As you inhale during this breathing exercise, imagine that your breath is guiding energy into every part of your body as if your breath and blood circulation are one.

1. Sit comfortably with your spine long.

2. Begin yogic breathing through your nose.

3. At the top of the inhale, hold your breath for 2 seconds without strain.

4. At the bottom of your exhale, hold your breath for 2 seconds.

5. Steps 3 and 4 comprise 1 round. Repeat for a total of 10 rounds. ◆

— THREE-SEAL BREATHING —

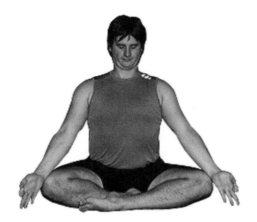

1. Sit in a comfortable cross-legged position on the floor with your spine long or sit in a chair with the back of the chair supporting your back.

2. Close your eyes. Breathe in and out through your nose.

3. As you inhale, contract your perineum by squeezing your anal sphincter to engage the root seal.

4. At the end of your inhale, draw your chin down 20 degrees and retract your head slightly so your ears align over your shoulders to engage the chin seal.

5. As you exhale, maintain both the root seal and the chin seal.

6. At the end of your exhalation, rapidly draw your belly in and up to engage the navel seal.

7. Inhale and release all three seals. Exhale naturally. ✦

YOUR NEXT MOVE

As with chapter 1, it's not necessary to master all the techniques and sequences in this chapter before moving on to chapter 3, which deals with the next kosha layer to be uncovered: meditation. Yogis devote their entire lives to gaining a greater understanding of the koshas through the practice of yoga, so don't expect to have each chapter all figured out before proceeding to the next; you don't want to take a lifetime to complete this book!

Once you get a sense of how the energy kosha ties into the postures and breathwork introduced in this chapter, you can begin to delve deeper into the layers of your consciousness by turning to the next chapter, on the meditation kosha.

CHAPTER 3

MEDITATION

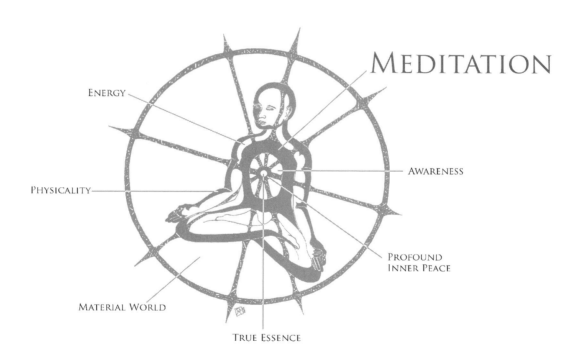

MEDITATION

ENERGY

PHYSICALITY

MATERIAL WORLD

TRUE ESSENCE

AWARENESS

PROFOUND
INNER PEACE

The next kosha to be uncovered in your journey toward inner peace is meditation. In this chapter, you'll start to closely examine your emotions and thought processes through the practice of meditation. This kosha will help you get in touch with what's going on in your heart and mind. The meditation kosha is an important layer to transcend because your emotions and thoughts serve to either further connect you to or disconnect you from your true self.

Simply put, positive thoughts lead to greater happiness, and negative thoughts trigger sadness, anger, and other difficult emotions. While there may be more to happiness than just positive thinking, that's where it really all begins.

You might know someone who appears to have it all—a well-paying job, fancy home, nice car, a healthy family—yet that person is perpetually cranky! This type of person is never quite content and always has something to complain about.

Then there's the individual who has little in the way of material goods but is upbeat and genuinely full of joy. Both examples reinforce my point: The thoughts you create about what's going on around you have a tremendous bearing on how you ultimately feel, and on how easily you can transcend the meditation kosha on your journey toward inner bliss.

THE POWER OF CHOICE

To understand the full extent of how the third kosha serves to benefit you, it's important to tease out the two types of thoughts you have every day: conscious and unconscious. On a conscious level, you *choose* to think one way or another—positively or negatively. Let's say your car starts sputtering and acting up. You take it to the mechanic, who says your car needs major repairs and you should expect to be without wheels for the next week. You can choose to perceive this news as negative or positive. Let's start with the negative. After all, it's pretty inconvenient not to have a car at your disposal. You'll have to rely on public transit, which means waking up extra early to get to the bus stop on time. Then you'll have to sit next to total strangers on a stuffy, crowded bus—if you're lucky enough to get a seat. Ugh!

Or, you could look at it another way. You won't have your car for a week, but while you're on the bus, you'll get to catch up on the novel you started months ago but haven't had time to finish at home. Plus, you get a break from dealing with rush hour traffic. Let the bus driver worry about the commute while you enjoy relaxing music on your MP3 player. Ahh, a chance to arrive at work feeling refreshed instead of frazzled.

See how one situation can produce two very different reactions depending on your thoughts? This underscores how powerful conscious thinking can be in altering your perception, your experiences, and ultimately your life.

UNDERSTANDING UNCONSCIOUS THOUGHTS

When it comes to unconscious thinking, you don't have the same power of choice. That's because unconscious thoughts—both negative and positive—are more ingrained. Consider, for example, your occupation in life. Perhaps you pursued a particular vocation because of deeply ingrained, unconscious ideas you have about yourself. These ideas might stem from your childhood. Take the case of Dana, a university professor who chose her line of work partly because her teachers and parents praised the high grades she received as a child. From an early age, Dana came to understand herself as being intelligent and successful at academics.

Let's change this scenario a bit and imagine that Dana's older brother received a lot of praise for the grades he got, while Dana received less praise even though her talent and skills were the same as in the first scenario. Because her brother gets the attention and accolades, Dana comes to believe that she isn't the true brain in the family, her brother is. These unconscious thoughts may keep Dana from pursuing a career in academics. Both examples illustrate how unconscious thinking feeds into self-perception. The issue here isn't whether academics is the right career for Dana; it's whether she chooses a career based on self-reflection and conscious thought, rather than unconscious thought and past influences that may not have much bearing on her desires and her current situation.

Meditation helps you bring the unconscious into the conscious, allowing you to choose one thought over another. This is an important process because it helps you create greater awareness of this kosha layer within yourself.

THE FEELING BODY

Thoughts on their own are just thoughts. What makes them especially powerful is their emotional impact. You don't just feel emotionally crummy out of nowhere. How could you? That unpleasant feeling was instigated by an unpleasant thought, conscious or unconscious. And just as your thoughts influence your feelings, your feelings influence your thoughts. When you have negative thoughts, you tend to feel bad, which makes you have more negative thoughts. Fortunately, the same is true of positive thoughts. Either way, think of it as a thought-emotion cycle. Once you have a clear sense of this relationship, you can more easily move through the meditation kosha layer.

Harnessing the power of your thoughts and emotions is where yoga's emphasis on a mind-body connection takes shape. Your mind represents thoughts, and your body represents emotions. To understand the physical manifestation of emotion, consider how your body feels when you're happy, when you're sad, and when you're angry. It's common to feel emotions in the gut (a gut instinct) or the heart (a broken heart).

Thoughts inform emotions, but it's easier to examine how you *feel* at any given moment than to constantly monitor every conscious thought that enters your head. Yet even to truly know how you feel requires a healthy relationship with your emotions. The meditation kosha is the gateway to that healthy relationship.

Once you can successfully tune in to your emotions, you can more readily allow positive thoughts into your conscious mind. You'll also begin to integrate difficult feelings into your life in a more meaningful way. This latter point may seem counterintuitive. Why would you want to integrate difficult feelings into your life? The purpose is to create a deeper understanding of why you behave the way you do. When this understanding becomes part of your consciousness, where the true power of choice lies, you bring yourself closer, kosha by kosha, to your true self.

ALL EMOTION IS GOOD

Most people would rather avoid unpleasant feelings, but all emotions are useful. It's healthy for humans to feel emotions, including difficult emotions. How we act on our emotions is what matters. For example, you might cope with emotions in a health-enhancing way or a health-destroying way. Let's say you're experiencing anger on a regular basis. Maybe it's over something to do with a coworker or tension at home between you and your partner. Whatever the trigger, it's the reaction you should be most concerned with. How you respond to that emotion can work in your favor, such as by sweating away your frustrations with a vigorous workout, or against you, perhaps by drowning your sorrows in one too many gin and tonics.

Many people live under the conscious or unconscious misconception that their thoughts and emotions are who they are. You might use self-imposed definitions to identify the essence of yourself, such as I'm an angry person, I'm a shy person, I'm a depressed person, or whatever comes to mind for you. In actuality, your true essence isn't a product of your thoughts and feelings. You are not your thoughts. You are not your feelings. Your true self is greater than any thought and any emotion. This realization is foundational to the meditation kosha.

With that in mind, it's important to recognize that tapping into your true essence isn't about being eternally elated. Endless happiness is hard to come by in today's society anyway. My hope is that you learn to strive for an *inner resilience*, where your thoughts are focused and your emotions are balanced. Meditation will help you achieve this goal.

Benefits of Healthy Emotional Awareness

When you're open to feeling your emotions and releasing blocked emotions, you're more likely to experience certain benefits:

- Increased creativity and imagination
- Increased feelings of wholeness, peace, tranquility, and love
- More internal and physical energy
- Deeper relationships with yourself and others
- An ability to be comfortable with the unknowableness of the future

QUIETING YOUR MIND WITH MEDITATION

As you've seen from previous chapters, physicality is one of yoga's main themes. Thousands of years ago, however, yoga's central premise was simply to still thoughts through meditation. Meditating quiets a busy mind, which allows you to seize greater control over your reactions to life. For example, when you quiet the running commentary in your brain, you gain some separation from ingrained beliefs you harbor about yourself and the world. Many people hold negative beliefs about themselves such as I'm dumb, I'm not athletic, I'm unattractive, or I'm timid. Through the process of meditation, your negative belief systems become less potent and wield less power over your ideas and your perceptions of yourself. Meditation is about letting go of the past in order to manifest the inherently positive benefits of being in the present.

The meditation practices in this chapter teach you how to begin transcending the meditation kosha by making your mind still, which simply means being aware and present in each moment. Although this may sound simple, it's actually very difficult for most of us. The easiest way to learn how to meditate is to focus on its overriding theme of being in the here and now. When you allow yourself—your mind—to be fully in the moment, there's no room for ruminating about what happened years ago or worrying about what needs to be accomplished tomorrow. This can be incredibly freeing and allows you to develop a consciousness where your thoughts naturally become more self-affirming and less self-debilitating. Being truly present can be elating.

The purpose of this chapter is to foster positive thoughts and emotions while freeing yourself from identification with negative thoughts. Through meditation, you'll begin to cultivate greater happiness as you energize this kosha layer and consciously choose a more positive outlook in life. You'll also learn how to become more aware of—and change, if need be—your unconscious beliefs. Some of these may serve you well in life; whereas others may inhibit you from moving beyond the meditation kosha toward true transcendence.

Benefits of Meditation

Here are just a few of the benefits of a meditative mind:

- Increased alertness and energy
- Greater clarity
- More compassion (when your mind stills, your heart opens)
- An ability to manifest your desires more efficiently
- A greater sense of presence, which leads to a calmer mind-body relationship
- Increased sensitivity to touch, taste, smell, sound, and sight

---

A BEGINNER'S WAY OF MEDITATING

Have you ever been in a situation where your thoughts were racing a mile a minute? Most of us have. Picture yourself sitting in a traffic jam and your cell phone has a dead battery. You're already late for a meeting or appointment, and you're becoming more agitated by the minute. You're worrying about how unimpressed your boss will be when you walk into the meeting late, or how flaky you'll look for showing up to an appointment behind schedule. These types of agitated thoughts tend to be unaware, unconscious, and frantic. In other words, you're not experiencing the world with a sense of mindfulness.

To turn this kind of situation into an experience that's mindful and meditative, simply slow down the commentary in your head. Here's how you do it:

1. **Breathe deeply,** focusing on long, slow exhalations. (Remember from chapter 2 that exhaling helps calm the mind and body.)

2. **Concentrate on something tangible,** like feeling your feet touching the ground. This focuses your mind and also instills grounding energy.

3. **Create space and silence** as best you can. Remove distractions. If possible, stop what's agitating you even if it's just for a moment. In the driving scenario above, you could briefly pull over to the side of the road.

The steps above lead to what I think of as a beginner's way of meditating. It's a simple practice anyone can employ, just about anywhere, to begin to develop a capacity to still the mind.

The next section explains how to take your meditative practice further using two distinct styles of meditation.

MEDITATION STYLES

Meditation helps you wake up to your thoughts and become aware of them, including how your thoughts affect your emotions and your body. When you're awake to the thought-emotion cycle, it will be easier for you to choose new thoughts that uplift your emotions. You can go about meditating in either an active way or a passive way. You'll find instructions for both active and passive meditation a bit later in the chapter. First, though, let's take a look at the purpose and benefits of each style.

ACTIVE MEDITATION

Active meditation is the easiest form of meditation for most people to get the hang of because it involves focusing your thoughts. The intention is to harness your thoughts into a state of singularity, or one-pointedness. You might already be familiar with this type of meditation, where you concentrate on one thing at a time, such as your breathing or where you gaze during yoga postures—or the candle gaze you learned in chapter 1. That technique is the first step to active meditation. As you practiced gazing at a candle flame for several minutes, you might have already begun to get a feel for meditation. Or, like many people, you might have noticed your mind wandering to this thought or that thought without any distinct direction. This chapter teaches you how to mentally zero in on a more meditative state.

When you engage in active meditation, your focus is singular, which serves to eliminate the negatives in your thinking. It's difficult to be bothered by worries or influenced by negative past impressions when your mind is pointed at the ebb and flow of your breathing or the flicker of a candle flame. The space in your mind is taken up by focus, and focus alone.

PASSIVE MEDITATION

Passive meditation is a more advanced version of meditating because it's so subtle. In active meditation, you actively point your mind. In passive meditation, you passively become a witness to your own consciousness. Think of it as looking at your inner layers for the purpose of becoming more self-aware. The goal is to observe your thoughts, tendencies, and patterns without judgment. When you're able to do this, you gain insight about the blueprint of who you are on the inside. The result is a broader perspective on your past impressions and ingrained beliefs, and who you've become as a result of your self-defining thoughts.

Passive meditation involves allowing thoughts to enter your mind like clouds floating in the sky. A thought floats in, and you become aware of that thought without reacting to it. Then you watch the thought drift by until the next thought comes onto the scene. There's a thought… There it goes… There's another thought… There it goes.

Compared to active meditation, your mind must be more still to practice passive meditation because it's so easy to get attached to a thought and become mentally sidetracked. This is natural, since most people spend a good deal of time paying attention to what's going on in their heads. The more you practice passive meditation, the easier it will become.

EVERYDAY OBSTACLES TO MEDITATION

On any given day you probably have a pretty decent excuse for why you can't make meditation happen. Modern society doesn't allow for much time to just sit quietly. In fact, in today's fast-paced world there doesn't seem to be any incentive to take a few moments to slow down, physically and mentally, and it may even be viewed as a waste of time. However, as you've begun to see in this chapter, slowing down through meditation has tremendous value, not only for your health and well-being, but also for your personal and spiritual transcendence.

That said, here are three common obstacles to meditation and tips for overcoming them:

Obstacle: Busyness with no space or downtime to retreat from your schedule.
Overcome it: You don't need tons of time to meditate. This may sound strange, but take a few extra moments in the washroom if that's all the alone time you can get. Another strategy is to set your alarm clock five or ten minutes earlier in the morning to carve out some time for yourself.

The Blank Mind Myth

Resist thinking of either active meditation or passive meditation as trying to achieve a clean slate in your head. Meditation is about cultivating a still mind, not a blank mind. When distracting thoughts come into your head, simply resist reacting to them. You can choose to give thoughts power or not.

It's sort of like a guy who keeps invading your space in hopes of getting your attention. If you ignore that person, he'll likely come back again and again, perhaps becoming more persistent for a while. But if he never receives your attention, he'll eventually give up. Thoughts that interrupt you during meditation are like that attention-seeker. Don't give them credence, and they'll stop coming around.

Obstacle: Too noisy.

Overcome it: You don't need complete silence while you meditate. True, the quieter, the better. But there's no need to hear a pin drop! Eliminate unwanted noise with earplugs or a white noise machine. Or use sound as part of your meditation by focusing on the sound of your breath, your hands clapping, or a chant. (Chapter 5 includes instructions for doing this.)

Obstacle: Feeling too scattered or restless to sit still.

Overcome it: Practice a sequence of yoga postures before you meditate to work some of the physical and mental restlessness out of your system. Begin with just a minute or two of meditation, and stick to active meditation versus passive meditation.

MEDITATION METHODS

This final section offers two methods for practicing meditation: an active meditation technique and a passive meditation technique. Here are a few tips to get you started:

- It's fine to practice both meditation styles in one day or even in one sitting. Just be sure to do the active meditation first.

- People who are extroverted, jumpy, or restless may find active meditation most rewarding. People who are introverted and naturally self-reflective may find passive meditation most comfortable.

- It's preferable to close your eyes as you meditate unless you're gazing at a candle flame or other object for active meditation. Closing your eyes allows your senses to withdraw to an inward dimension.

- Try to bookend your day with meditation, practicing for about five minutes at both the beginning and the end of your day. Meditating in the morning instills a positive intention and tone for the day. Meditating in the evening or before bed sets a nice tone for sleeping.

- As you become more familiar with meditation, work your way up to ten minutes per practice.

Five Seated Postures for Active and Passive Meditation

Choose one of the five yoga-style seated postures below for your meditation practice. They're arranged in order from easiest to most advanced. Begin with the first option below (Seated Cross-Legged) and work your way up to the most complex (Full Lotus). You may also meditate while sitting in a chair if you prefer.

In any of the seated postures, your knees should be lower than the top of your hip bones. If your level of flexibility doesn't allow you to achieve this position, sit on a yoga bolster, a meditation cushion, or even two or three folded blankets.

You shouldn't feel knee tension in any of the seated postures below. When moving your legs manually to get into or out of a pose, draw awareness to dropping your knees and externally rotating your hips throughout the movement. To protect your knee joints, your thighs should be rotating externally toward the floor.

Regarding hand position, there are two recommendations: The first is to place your hands on your knees, palms down, with the tip of your thumb and the tip of your index finger touching. This position is good for grounding. The second is to place the back of your hands on your knees with the tip of your thumb and the tip of your index finger touching and your palms facing up toward the sky. This position is good for receiving energy.

Finally, be sure to change your leg position with each meditation session so that neither your right leg nor your left is always on the top.

— Seated Cross-Legged Pose —

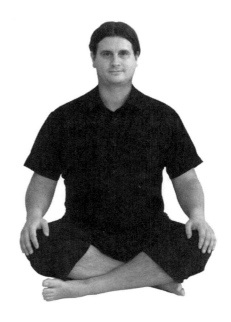

1. Sit in a natural cross-legged position, with your left leg in front of your right leg or your right leg in front of your left leg.

2. Hold your spine long and either keep your chin parallel to the floor or tuck it down slightly.

3. Switch which leg is in front for each new meditation session. ✦

— Beginner Accomplished Pose —

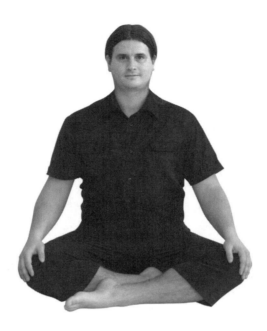

1. Begin in the **Seated Cross-Legged** position.

2. Bring your right heel slightly to the left of the midline of your body and your left heel slightly to the right of the midline of your body with the outside edge of both feet on the floor. Either foot can be in front, and both should be as close to your groin as possible. Press your thighs toward the floor.

3. Hold your spine long and either keep your chin parallel to the floor or tuck it down slightly.

4. Switch which leg is in front for each new meditation session. ✦

— Intermediate Accomplished Pose —

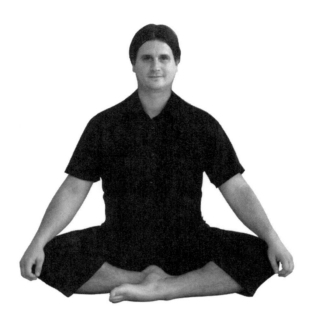

1. Begin in the **Seated Cross-Legged** position.

2. Place both heels at the midline of your body on the floor. One heel should be in front of the other, with the outside edge of both feet on the floor. Either foot can be in front, and both should be as close to the middle of your pelvis as possible. If your thighs aren't in contact with the floor, stick with **Beginner Accomplished Pose** until you have greater flexibility.

3. Hold your spine upright and long and either keep your chin parallel to the floor or tuck it down slightly.

4. Switch which leg is in front for each new meditation session. ◆

— HALF LOTUS —

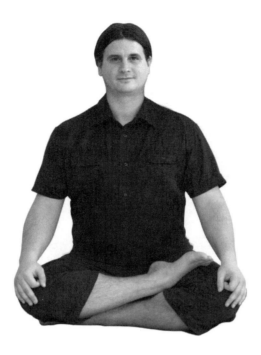

1. Begin in the **Seated Cross-Legged** position.

2. Use your hands to place your right heel at the crease of your left hip flexor. This is where the upper leg bends at the hip. To protect your knee, the toes on your right foot should be curling toward your knee. Your left heel should naturally be close to your right sit bone.

3. Hold your spine upright and long and either keep your chin parallel to the floor or tuck it down slightly.

4. Switch legs for each new meditation session. ◆

— Full Lotus —

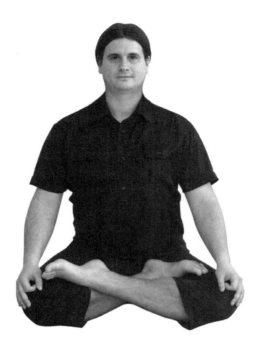

1. Begin in **Half Lotus** with your right heel at the crease of your left hip flexor.

2. Use your hands to place your left leg over your right leg and position your left heel at the crease of your right hip flexor. To protect your knees, curl the toes on each foot toward the knee of that same leg.

3. Hold your spine upright and long and either keep your chin parallel to the floor or tuck it down slightly.

4. Switch legs for each new meditation session. ◆

— ACTIVE MEDITATION METHOD —

1. Sit comfortably with your spine long in one of the five positions above, or in a chair.

2. Point your mind by focusing on your breath as you inhale and exhale naturally using yogic breathing through your nose. Other options for the focus in active meditation include fixing your gaze on a candle flame or a black dot on a white piece of paper. ◆

Another active meditation approach is beginner japa yoga meditation—a precursor to a technique you'll learn in chapter 5: Sitting in one of the postures described already, begin clapping your hands. Point your mind toward the physical feeling of your hands touching each other. Then combine your focus on both the touch sensation and the sound of the clapping. You may find that changing the speed at which you clap helps you maintain the best focus.

— PASSIVE MEDITATION METHOD —

1. Sit comfortably with your spine long in one of the five positions already described, or in a chair.

2. Hold your body as still as you can and use your mind's eye to watch your thoughts. Allow each thought to drift through your mind without judgment or reaction. Simply witness the thought or feeling.

3. Return over and over to the present moment without actually focusing on anything in particular. ◆

SIT QUIETLY WITH A QUIET MIND

Meditation allows you to peel back the layer of yourself that's concerned with your mental and emotional processes. You must be able to reflect on the state of your thoughts and feelings, as you learned to do in this chapter, before you can fully explore the fourth kosha, which is concerned with your sense of personal awareness. I recommend that you devote some time to practicing meditation before delving too deeply into the next chapter. And once you do start working ahead, please continue with the meditation methods in this chapter, as well.

Meditation is so easy to implement, and it brings such great rewards. It truly is one of the keys to inner bliss. When done often enough, meditation can help you better understand and appreciate your inner sensibilities and kosha layers. All it takes to effect lifelong change in a positive and profound direction is a few minutes a day of sitting quietly with a quiet mind.

CHAPTER 4

AWARENESS

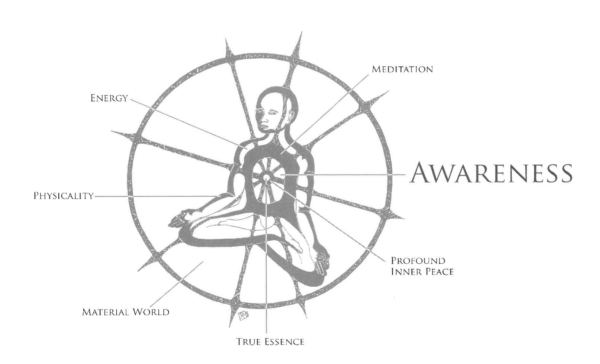

This chapter will help you develop a more holistic connection to yourself through the yogic process of living from within. By developing your fourth kosha, the awareness kosha, you'll increase your ability to live from within and honor your truest wants and needs so you can experience greater personal satisfaction in both inner and outer dimensions.

This chapter will help you explore the importance of your own inner wisdom for problem solving, finding your life's passion and joy, and opening to creativity. The intention is to cultivate a lifestyle that feels most right and meaningful to you.

MANIFESTING YOUR DESIRES

Have you ever heard a story about someone who's steered his or her life in an entirely new direction or taken an incredible leap of faith? These stories usually involve people who have developed a strong sense of awareness about themselves.

There's the high-powered lawyer who walks away from security and wealth to run a modest bed-and-breakfast in the quiet countryside. Or it might be the timid fifty-year-old who's been strumming a guitar in the basement for years and finally drums up the courage to join a rock band and play live gigs.

What makes certain people decide their current path in life no longer serves them? How come some people pursue their dreams even if it scares the daylights out of them? The purpose of this chapter is to answer these questions in the framework of the fourth yogic kosha: awareness. Through the course of this chapter, you'll become familiar with how your awareness kosha can guide and create your life path.

INCREASING PERSONAL AWARENESS THROUGH YOGA

Creating a clear and strong connection to your innermost needs and desires is and always has been a major tenet in yogic philosophy and practice. The intention of this yoga-centered book is to assist you in gaining insight about the meaning of *your* life through an understanding of the koshas. As you delve deeper into each kosha layer, you open the door to a more blissful existence. Thus far you've worked with the physicality, energy, and meditation koshas. The awareness kosha explained in this chapter is another step toward identifying and living your bliss.

Let me clarify that while a deeper sense of personal awareness might assist you in setting out on a new career path or deciding whether to start a family, it can also inform something of less magnitude, such as choosing your next creative project or vacation spot.

Although the awareness kosha can help you set goals toward getting or becoming what you wish for in the material world, material success is only one dimension of manifesting your desires. Your inner wisdom (another way to describe the awareness kosha) is equally concerned with less tangible processes, such as healing yourself emotionally, restoring depleted energy, or cultivating stronger love relationships. The awareness kosha encompasses the gamut of life's experiences, big and small.

USING AWARENESS TO MAP YOUR LIFE'S PATH

A lot of people confuse awareness or inner wisdom with intuition, even though they aren't entirely the same thing. I would describe awareness as a form of deeper intuition. However, I urge you to separate inner wisdom from the common conception of intuition as simply instinctive knowing or a flash of insight. Awareness is a more active process and involves listening for deeper messages in order to gain a profound understanding of yourself. It's about really knowing who you are and being attuned to the subtler aspects of yourself.

I like to think of awareness as a perfect balance between destiny and free will. Here, I use "destiny" in the sense of your life's calling, what you were meant to do and accomplish in your lifetime. Destiny is connected to a higher power—call it God, Buddha, Atman, the universe, or whatever feels most comfortable for you. Free will, on the other hand, is the actions you choose to take based on your passions, skills, talents, interests, and opportunities. For example, you might have the physiology and prowess of a world-class athlete, but if you don't exert your will to pursue and nurture that aspect of yourself, you'll never live out that destiny.

Tapping into the fourth kosha, the layer of yourself that's concerned with awareness, means gaining a better sense of how to proceed in each moment. But it's also about the bigger picture. The greater your awareness, the easier it becomes to take the right steps on your soul's evolutionary path. Think of awareness as a guidance system, an internal compass, toward your fullest potential in life—your truest self.

COMING BACK TO YOUR INNER WISDOM

Awareness has always been in you. Like all the koshas, it's innate. You might remember having a keen sense of awareness as a child. Kids dream big, don't they? And they're pretty attuned to what interests them and what doesn't. If you've ever been to a young child's birthday party, you might know what I mean. Here's the scene: The child tears open all of the gifts, then makes a beeline for the one or two that he or she likes best. There's no going through the motions to please all of the gift givers and show appreciation for everything received. Young kids know what they're most interested in, and they devote their attention to those things.

As kids get older, they still have that inner wisdom about what they want and don't want, but they may begin to dismiss it in response to external pressures. Take ten-year-old Deanne. She has her heart set on joining a soccer team, but her parents enroll her in ballet lessons instead. Deanne might agree to ballet, but she's putting on a show to please her parents. On the inside, she's pretty aware about what feels like the best fit for her (soccer!).

Think back to your own childhood. When did you feel your own inner wisdom? It might have been a sureness about something you wanted at that stage in your life. What's that awareness like now that you're an adult? If you feel as if you've lost it, this chapter will help you get in touch with this sacred kosha layer once again.

Looking Inward for Fulfillment

Unfortunately, for lots of adults internal wisdom tends to go numb, and for some it shuts down altogether. You might feel that in some ways you've become a master at living in denial—perhaps not in all aspects of your life, but some. Through years of doing what others expect or want you to do, you may have lost touch with your awareness kosha. You no longer access that place inside you because you've essentially forgotten it was there.

Take the example of a college-aged man named Alan. His great-grandfather was a doctor. His grandfather was a doctor. His father is a doctor, and so is his mother. Guess what the family's expectation is for Alan? To become a doctor, of course. He obliges but experiences a terrible sense of uneasiness during med school. This could be seen as a failing or weakness, but actually it's his deeper wisdom sending him a message: "Alan, you don't want to be a doctor."

Like Alan, you might lose touch with your awareness kosha because of pressures from family and friends. Or this disconnection might be a product of pressure from society in general. Media messages, technology, and fast-paced living typically do more to pull you away from your inner wisdom than toward it. One clear example is how so many people spend so little time being by themselves these days. Everywhere you go, people are chatting on cell phones, checking digital devices, and surfing the Internet. Few people seem to be engaging in personal reflection anymore. If this technologically oriented, overly connected lifestyle sounds like you, consider that one of the easiest ways to tap into your deeper awareness is simply to stop distracting yourself all of the time. Unplug from technology more often to access what's in your heart.

The Side Effects of Accessing (or Not Accessing) Awareness

When you're successfully accessing the awareness kosha, you're likely to feel heightened creativity, imagination, playfulness, joy, ease, presence—qualities you might also use to describe the happy state of being a child. On the other hand, if you perpetually block your deeper awareness, you'll have a tough, if not impossible, time transcending toward your true essence. At first you might feel unfulfilled and find yourself just coping, getting by, and barely making it from day to day. That sense of unfulfillment may eventually intensify to feelings of despair, anxiety, worry, dread, hopelessness, depression, or any number of other unpleasant struggles.

Sometimes people don't access the awareness kosha because they simply don't know it's there. But you can also ignore this kosha on purpose. Given that the awareness kosha is one key to unlocking inner bliss, you might wonder why anyone would choose to block it out. The answer is fear. In fact, fear is an emotion some people actually confuse with awareness.

FEAR VERSUS AWARENESS

At the start of this chapter, I gave a couple of examples of people who followed a passion despite the trepidation that might have come with it. Sometimes listening to your inner voice stirs up feelings of discomfort even if it's pointing you in a direction you ultimately want to go. Because of this, you may have a tough time differentiating between fearful thoughts and communication from your wisdom center. Both can send messages about how to act in a given situation or about the big picture of your life. So how do you know if that voice inside is coming from a place of inner wisdom or a place of fear and resistance?

The simplest way I can describe it is this: When you act out of fear, you probably aren't very present in the moment, the here and now. Fear is attached to thoughts and emotions of the past (something that's scared you before) or the future (something you're afraid might happen). Communication from a place of complete awareness is characterized by present-moment awareness. It's also neutral. It's a response to your life's circumstance based on compassion for yourself versus a reaction born out of a fight, flight, or freeze instinct.

I'll give you an example of how this might play out. Imagine a woman who has a beautiful singing voice but suffers from a very common fear: speaking and performing in public. Her passion is singing and she yearns to be a musician, but her inner voice says, "Don't dream too big. You're not cut out to be a singer." Is that voice coming from her wisdom center, or a place of fear? You can identify it as fear because the awareness kosha is always self-nurturing and self-supportive. If you experience doubt or confusion, or if you lack a sense of worthiness about a decision or course in life, you're being driven by something other than your wisdom center. Following a path of true self-awareness will always benefit you, even if it scares you, too.

The important thing is to act on the awareness you gain about yourself. This is how you come to a place of greater self-acceptance and happiness. It's entirely possible to set your sights on a life's passion, goal, or intention then hide behind the process of preparing for that goal versus moving in a direction toward actually reaching that goal. An example is someone who enrolls in one self-help workshop after another without ever making meaningful changes. I call this being stuck at the point of intention. You might tell yourself what you hope to accomplish: I intend to rest more, I want to focus my creativity, I'm going to react with less anger. However, the emphasis remains on the intention to pursue the goal rather than acting toward the goal itself.

Tuning in to your awareness kosha is half of the equation. The other half is figuring out what to do with your inner wisdom once you access it. The rest of this chapter zeroes in on this vital integration of awareness and action. You'll learn how to listen to your deeper awareness, and then act on what you uncover.

INTEGRATION METHODS

Manifesting what you desire in life involves three steps:

- **Step 1: Establish an awareness of what you want.** The awareness meditation technique described below will help you accomplish this step.

- **Step 2: Create intention for change.** With this step, you begin to bridge your internal awareness to your outer life.

- **Step 3: Channel intention into action.** You may choose to continue down a path you're on if it's positive. Or you may act on transforming something old, such as a behavioral or mental habit that doesn't nurture you, into something new.

STEP 1: ESTABLISH AN AWARENESS OF WHAT YOU WANT

As you learned in chapter 3, meditation is foundational to yogic living. You'll use the following Awareness Meditation to begin the three-step process outlined above. This meditation technique will help you open mental and emotional doors to your awareness center and connect to your inner voice of awareness. The best way to think about communicating with your wisdom center is like this: If your heart or your gut were to speak to you, what would those deeper intuition centers be saying to you?

As you meditate, try to avoid choosing an area of your life to focus on, such as relationships or career. Let your wisdom center steer you. In other words, get out of your own way and allow the process to just happen. Listening to your inner voice involves surrendering control over the practice.

— AWARENESS MEDITATION —

Here are a few guidelines to keep in mind as you do the Awareness Meditation:

- You may do this meditation at any time of day. However, meditating in the morning or evening is an especially nice way to start or end the day.

- It's fine to do this meditation every day if it feels right for you.

- Read through the instructions a few times so that you can do the entire meditation without referring to the text.

Do the meditation described below three times, changing your physical position each time. The first time, use the Relaxation Pose; the second time, use Child's Pose; and the third time, use the Beginner Accomplished Pose. Each posture helps you access your inner wisdom from a different perspective. You should be familiar with these three poses by now and the illustrations below will refresh your memory. If need be, refer back to chapters 1 and 3 for details on each posture.

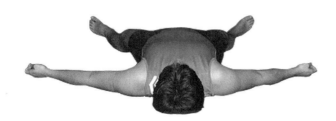

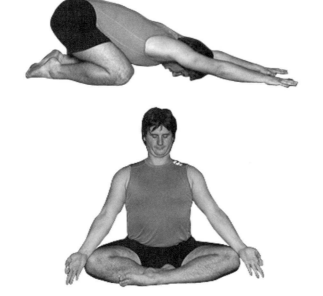

1. Find a place with few or no distractions.

2. Get into the **Relaxation Pose** and close your eyes.

3. Begin ujjayi breathing as described in chapter 1, inhaling and exhaling slowly through your nose and breathing deeply, into your lower belly.

4. Focus your internal gaze at your heart or your navel. You may discover that one of these areas helps you tap into your internal awareness more than the other. Experiment with both to find what works best for you.

5. Open yourself to your inner place of knowing, where you receive moment insights—messages that arise during the course of your meditation. You'll find that the most pressing insights start to become most apparent.

6. Continue meditating from your awareness center for about 5 minutes.

7. Repeat the meditation while in **Child's Pose**, again meditating for about 5 minutes.

8. Repeat the meditation once again, this time in **Beginner Accomplished Pose**, and again meditating for about 5 minutes. ✦

STEP 2: CREATE INTENTION FOR CHANGE

Out of your awareness meditation, you probably noticed one or more underlying themes. Your next step is to determine how to bring that deeper awareness into your life so you begin or continue to live in accordance with your inner wisdom. How will change show up in your life? What are your intentions for moving forward? Think of intentions as goal setting: coming up with practical steps you can take to alter or enhance one or more aspects of your life. For example, perhaps your wisdom center is pointing you in the direction of a more energetic existence. Right now, you feel so tired at the end of the day, your productivity and creativity is at a near standstill. Three intentions for generating more energy might be going to bed one hour earlier at night; reserving some time each morning for a brisk walk, which will help you lose a bit of weight and stimulate your energy; and devising a gradual exit strategy to remove yourself from a time-consuming career commitment you no longer enjoy.

— VISUALIZATION EXERCISE —

Here's a visualization technique that will help bring your inner wisdom into your life through intention:

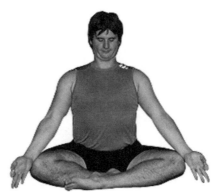

1. Sit quietly in any of the seated postures outlined in chapter 3: **Seated Cross-Legged Pose, Beginner Accomplished Pose, Intermediate Accomplished Pose, Half Lotus, Full Lotus,** or in a chair with your back supported. (If you sit cross-legged, remember to ensure that your knees are below the top of your hip bones. If necessary, sit on a cushion or yoga bolster to achieve this position.) Close your eyes.

2. Visualize yourself acting out your intentions. This means visualizing yourself in action, not visualizing the end result of those actions. The outcome isn't all that important. It's the process that matters.

3. Include all of your senses in the visualization. As you imagine enacting your intentions, what do you see, hear, feel, smell, and taste?

4. Once you've visualized yourself in action, let the mental imagery go and come back to the present moment. You've put the intention out there. For transformation to truly occur, now you must act on your intention. ◆

In the example above, the end result would be having more energy because of getting more sleep each night, getting active and losing a bit of weight, and creating more time for yourself. Visualizing the intention in this example means imagining going to bed when the clock says 9:30 p.m., walking at a fast pace around your neighborhood, or delegating some part of your job to others.

Using this same example, what would it look like to include all your senses in the visualization? When you're going to bed, what does your pillow feel like on your cheek? As you walk around your neighborhood, how does the morning air smell? When delegating tasks to others, what sounds are in the environment around you?

STEP 3: CHANNEL INTENTION INTO ACTION

This is the point at which you roll up your sleeves and get to work, so to speak. At this stage, you must actually do what you imagined during the visualization exercise in step 2. In other words, hold yourself accountable to acting on your intentions. One way to do this is by looking back. Acknowledge what you've already accomplished to inspire yourself, and also to help redefine your goals if necessary. How have you propelled yourself toward greater transformation? What worked for you? What didn't? Continuing with the example above, maybe a morning walk and delegating some tasks at work were effective in terms of boosting your energy and going to bed early wasn't. That's fine; not every potential solution will work. If you act on your intentions and determine a specific action wasn't entirely effective, it's okay to reassess your intention or replace it with a new one.

Here are two other suggestions for accountability. If they work for you, great. If not, experiment with other techniques to find an approach that will help you stay accountable:

1. **Journaling.** Record your intentions, perhaps one per page. For each, make a daily record of the concrete steps you took to honor the intention. Then go back and review your patterns and progress often.

2. **Enlist a friend.** Some people have a hard time being accountable to themselves. If you're inclined to let yourself off the hook, ask a trusted friend to help you stay the course. Tell your friend what you want to accomplish and how you plan to do it, and be sure to set up a plan for how your friend will keep you accountable. For example, your friend might call you on a regular basis to ask about your progress, or he or she might even participate in your action steps.

THE SACREDNESS OF INNER KNOWING

Once you come to the sacred place of greater inner knowing, you'll be in a position to direct yourself and your life in the most useful and satisfying ways possible. As with the other three kosha layers I've discussed so far, developing and transcending the awareness kosha is a never-ending process. You must engage in the practices in this chapter on an ongoing basis. After all, life is meant to be a series of new awarenesses and transformative experiences.

Hopefully this chapter has helped you rekindle or further ignite your connection to your wisdom center. Now I invite you to fan that fire by reading the next chapter, on the fifth and final kosha—profound inner peace.

CHAPTER 5

PROFOUND INNER PEACE

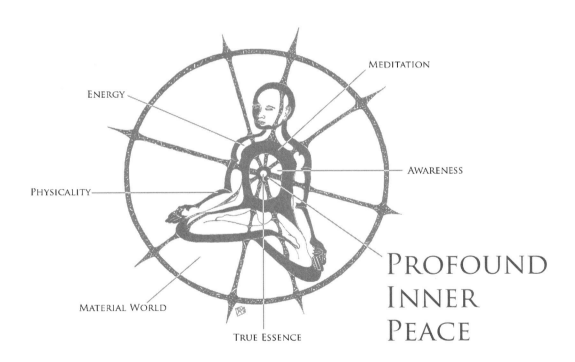

The practices in the first four chapters of this book have led you through an exploration of the first four koshas: physicality, energy, meditation, and awareness. Hopefully this has helped you develop a more positive and powerful sense of self on physical, mental, and emotional levels. As part of this process, you've begun shedding external influences and stressors that have been clouding your inner sensitivities. Everything you've read in this book so far has been leading you to a more meaningful understanding of your higher self so that your inner light can shine more brightly through each kosha layer.

This chapter covers the fifth and innermost kosha: profound inner peace. This is the deepest kosha layer and closely surrounds your true essence, or Atman. The focus of this spiritually rooted kosha is the celebration of joy, bliss, and love. These feelings go beyond simple emotions. They are states of being: joy and bliss in life, and all-encompassing love for self and others.

By the time you reach this subtlest of kosha layers, much of the hard work has been done. Looking back to chapter 1, you learned to cleanse and strengthen the first kosha, physicality, through purification practices and the asanas. In chapter 2, you explored the second kosha, energy, to create unobstructed prana flows in your body. In chapter 3, you turned to stilling and focusing your mind in an exploration of the third kosha, meditation. In chapter 4, you journeyed into the fourth kosha, awareness, to gain deeper insight about how to live from within. Now you stand at the threshold of the celebratory realm of genuine joy and bliss. It's time to reap the natural rewards of everything you've accomplished.

JOY FROM WITHIN

Profound inner peace can be felt anywhere, anytime. However, modern life doesn't typically support the bliss body (another way of saying profound inner peace). In the modern world, life is often too rushed, stressful, and packed to the gills. As a result, most people overlook the experience of joyous celebration simply for its own sake.

The good news is, you can make profound inner peace a more prominent part of your everyday life. By creating a healthier relationship with your first four kosha layers using the concepts and tangible steps in this book, the expression of profound inner peace will come more readily. That said, you can catch glimpses of intense elation at any time in your life. You may be able to recall instances when this happened to you, perhaps a sensation of deep joy from watching your child absorbed in play, or a sense of bliss from a good flow during your asana practice. Profound inner peace is possible even in the simplest and subtlest of moments.

In fact, it's often the times we least expect profound inner peace to appear that it does. When you have an expectation about what's supposed to make you happy, your mind will have a strong attachment to some sort of result—and you may feel disappointment if this doesn't occur. When you let go of attachment to specific results or outcomes, you make way for the profound inner peace you may find in whatever comes to pass.

Many people get wound up in knots planning occasions that they anticipate will be blissful, such as a holiday or a wedding. The beautiful thing about profound inner peace, though, is that it can't be planned. It just is. Whether it's a fleeting feeling or joy that lasts all day, knowing a place of inner peace comes largely from being present in the here and now. Through development, and ultimately transcendence, of your koshas, you have the power to multiply and extend these moments so they appear in your life more frequently and with greater magnitude.

INNER PEACE IS YOUR BIRTHRIGHT

Profound inner peace is always there; you're just more or less aware of it depending on how much the fifth kosha sheath masks or doesn't mask your true essence. In fact, even an initial realization that you aren't happy with your life or aspects of your life is a step toward inner peace because it means you're finally shedding the cloaks of denial that dim your inner light. Consider this concept: It's your birthright to be joyous. It expresses who you really are. The idea that you were meant to experience profound inner peace might seem strange, because blissfulness isn't a familiar feeling for many people.

One reason the bliss body feels foreign in modern times is because so many people seek "peace" or "bliss" through material things or circumstances: If I can just get that job, lose some weight, find a partner, earn more money (or whatever), I'll be happy. Of course, none of this is related to profound inner peace. Circumstances don't bring you inner peace. Rather, the circumstances you find yourself in reflect your sense of inner peace. Profound inner peace opens the door to those paths in life that bring you optimal satisfaction, love, and joy. When a sacred peace is present, your choices and actions come from a pure place—a place that's concerned with what's best for you and your capacity to serve others.

IDENTIFYING PROFOUND INNER PEACE

You might be wondering how to know when you're experiencing a healthy relationship with your fifth kosha layer. Is it a good mood? The bliss body can put you in a good mood, but it's not about a mood per se. It's joy that radiates from within.

Profound inner peace is rooted in sacredness and spirituality—in a closer connection between your inner self and Atman. When profound inner peace is present, you have a greater sense of creativity and abundance and feel a deeper intimacy in relationships. You feel as if you're living fully in your life's vocation. There's energy, laughter, and humor. There's lightness—and ecstasy. You feel comfortable going with the flow of life versus feeling attached to outcomes, worried about the past or future, or influenced by external factors, such as others' expectations. Profound inner peace celebrates life and self.

There is one important caveat: Profound inner peace doesn't eradicate all negative feelings and frustrating times. You're human, after all. Nothing in this book or in yogic philosophy promises unrelenting joy every minute of every day. You may feel as if you're struggling at times in your life, but it doesn't mean you can't access profound inner peace. The idea is to work toward experiencing bliss as a predominant theme in your life. Sure, off-putting thoughts, feelings, and situations may arise even when you're strongly connected to inner peace. The difference is that they don't dramatically alter your day or disposition.

SERVING YOURSELF BY SERVING OTHERS

Another beautiful aspect of profound inner peace is its capacity to expand without effort. As you cultivate inner peace, you'll find yourself drawn to serve others. You'll feel an impulse to give to and help those around you. I like to think of this as a natural law of the universe: Abundance begets abundance. When you experience bliss, you want to express and share that bliss with others, which in turn creates even more bliss. Think of a time when helping someone else enhanced your good feelings and positive energy. When you spread joy, it comes back to you. By giving to others, you give to yourself. It's an age-old concept that remains meaningful in the modern world.

Serving others might involve helping out in a charitable sense. However, I'm also talking about contributing to a deeper collective unconscious, where positive energy naturally builds on itself. Here's an example. Harold is a man with a rotten disposition. He scowls at others, makes snide remarks, and cuts people off in traffic. Harold is spreading his negative energy and uneasiness around. Of course, a kinder, friendlier person would spread positive energy; however, that's not the point I want to make here.

Let's say that grouchy old Harold encounters Maria, who's operating from an inner place of balance, groundedness, and compassion. She's impervious to Harold's rudeness and social dis-ease. Maria doesn't react to his meanness; she smiles. She responds with kindness and compassion. By doing so, Maria reflects to Harold just how unpleasant his behavior is. Harold is used to having people mirror his negative energy, but when Maria's reaction is the opposite, Harold sees himself more clearly. Through this awareness, he learns to lighten up.

CREATIVITY FLOWS NATURALLY

Another benefit of enjoying a strong connection to your peace center is feeling a natural flow of creativity. Artists who seek transcendence and access their inner peace find heightened inspiration in their creative endeavors. If you think this doesn't apply to you, be aware that creativity isn't limited to the fine arts. For accountants, playing with numbers can be creative. Lawyers engage in the art of negotiating. Teachers may bring a great deal of creativity to bear in preparing lesson plans. Occupations aside, planning a vacation, finding ways to entertain your kids, decorating your home, or even just cooking a meal are also ways to express the inspiration that flows from inner peace. And yoga, too, provides a canvas for expressing creativity. The practical approaches below will help you begin to express your creativity through the art of yoga.

METHODS FOR CELEBRATING BLISS

In exploring your fifth kosha, or bliss body, the practice of yoga takes a turn toward sound and music. The methods you'll learn below can express your inner elation. Alternatively, they can assist you in reaching profound inner peace if this aspect of yourself requires a bit of coaxing to be fully realized.

You may find that the practices below provide that final push or tangible guidance you need to get a taste of profound inner peace.

In the remainder of this chapter, you'll learn two forms of practice for developing your bliss body and enhancing its growth. One is to repeat a mantra through the practice of a spiritual discipline called *japa yoga*. The Sanskrit word *japa* means "to utter or repeat internally." Reciting the mantra described below allows you to meditate on sound as a way to encourage self-realization. This active meditation on sound is especially good for maintaining mental concentration; when your brain is absorbed in making sound, it's less likely to wander or get caught up in your other senses.

Japa yoga also prepares you for the second method of enhancing your inner peace I'll describe: *kirtan*, a call-and-response expression of *nada yoga*. *Nada* means "sound" in Sanskrit, so you can think of nada yoga as leading you to a transformative place through sound and tone. In both sacred and melodic senses, sound is a form of celebration, and this is where the practice of kirtan comes in.

Mala Beads

Some people use a string of japa mala beads in conjunction with this japa yoga recitation. You can find mala beads at many new age stores or shops where yoga equipment is sold.

Hold the bead next to the string's knot between your thumb and middle finger on your right hand only. Each time you recite the mantra, use your right thumb to move to the next bead. After you've touched all of the beads on the string and have come to the other end of the knot, reverse direction and continue repeating the mantra until you reach the knot one last time.

— JAPA YOGA —

For japa yoga practice, you'll repeat the Sanskrit mantra *Om Namah Shivaya* in three different ways: saying it aloud, whispering it, and then reciting it mentally. You may do this every day as part of your main practice if it feels right to do so. If you like, visit my website (www.wadeimremorissette.com) and download an hour-long MP3 audio file of the *Om Namah Shivaya* mantra accompanied by rhythmic guitar. The downloadable file is available for free or by donation.

Before we get into the detailed method, let's take a look at what this mantra means. Translated literally, *Om* means "universal sound," *Namah* means "give reverence to," and *Shivaya* refers to Shiva, the Hindu god of destruction and renewal. While a literal translation would be along the lines of "I bow to Shiva," the intent, as I see it, is "Letting go of the old; consciously bringing in the new."

1. Sit comfortably with your spine long in any of the five seated meditation poses described in chapter 3, or sit in a chair if you prefer.

2. Repeat *Om Namah Shivaya* using the following sequence, from easiest to do to most subtle. You may repeat the mantra quickly or slowly; there's no set speed for doing so. However, you may find that a faster pace helps you maintain mental focus more easily.

1. *Vaikhari.* The easiest method, this involves speaking aloud at a normal volume. Repeat the mantra for 2 minutes using vaikhari.
2. *Upamsu.* The intermediate method, this involves whispering. Repeat the mantra for 2 minutes using upamsu.
3. *Manasika.* The subtlest method, this involves silent, mental recitation. Repeat the mantra for 2 minutes using manasika.

3. Reverse the order of the sequence above, continuing with manasika for 2 minutes, then returning to upamsu for 2 minutes, and ending with vaikhari for 2 minutes.

4. End the practice by chanting "om" once, as in the Clarity Breath in chapter 2. ✦

Alternatively, you may also repeat the *Om Namah Shivaya* mantra through writing. This method is called *likhita*.

— KIRTAN —

When you repeat a mantra in private, you're doing japa yoga; when it's done to music in a community of others, it's an expression of nada yoga known as kirtan. Kirtan is the melodic expression of communal celebration based on a call-and-response chant. A lead vocalist—called a *wallah* (male) or *walli* (female)—sings a mantra that the audience then repeats back. Because kirtan involves melodies, music, and instruments familiar to Westerners, you may find it a more accessible way to enjoy meditating on sound. Plus, music is so universal that it often transcends cultural boundaries.

There are two ways for you to participate in this yogic practice: Find a kirtan gathering or concert in your area, or play a kirtan CD and repeat the words of the wallah or walli. Kirtan CDs are available through Nutone Music (www.nutonemusic.com).

INVITE HAPPINESS INTO YOUR INNER WORLD

Developing the spiritual sheath of profound inner peace is the fifth key to unlocking your inner bliss. However, in order to settle into this sacred place we all possess, you must open yourself to pure happiness. Inviting unbridled bliss into your inner world prepares you for the complete emergence of your inherent true essence.

CHAPTER 6

INTEGRATING YOUR TRUE ESSENCE INTO THE OUTER WORLD

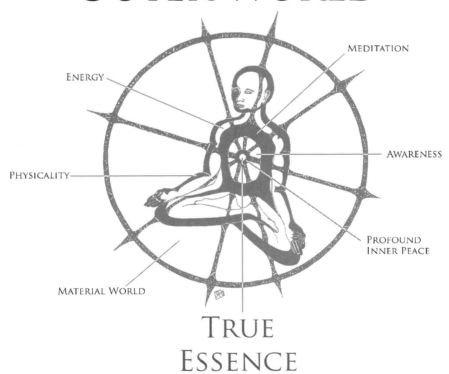

In this final chapter, it's time to flesh out the meaning and significance of drawing closer to the true essence of yourself—what I have been referring to throughout this book as Atman. This chapter is the culmination of everything you've learned in *Transformative Yoga*. Purifying the five koshas has been the key to unlocking the inner bliss of knowing your true essence, or Atman.

I want to be clear that Atman has always been with you. It's an unwavering, immortal spirit. It was present when you were born, and before that. It will be there until you die, and after that. You may recall that in the introduction I said you can't live in the world of Atman all the time. However, you can create a stronger tie or connection to Atman, similar to how a fetus is attached to its mother and nourished by an umbilical cord.

Atman is a yogic interpretation of God. The word "Atman" isn't universally known; however, the concept of Atman is widely recognized. What I call Atman, various religions might interpret as God, Allah, or Buddha, to name a few. However, I want to firmly establish that this book is not about religion. Yoga is a practice and a science, not a religion. Like previous chapters, this chapter deals with the yogic tradition of self-exploration and personal transcendence. Even so, while the approach in this book isn't intended to be or replace religious doctrine, belief, or practice, it does work on the assumption that something greater than ourselves exists.

MAKING SENSE OF THE INDESCRIBABLE

True essence is a formless spirit, so it's impossible to sum it up in a neat definition or even satisfactorily describe it. If—through faith—you believe Atman exists, that's good enough. And that's why you do the work laid out in this book: to draw yourself nearer to your true essence.

Some people are more closely connected to their true essence than others. However, I believe Atman exists to the same degree in all of us regardless of outer differences. If you believe in Atman, you accept the notion that everyone possesses the same spiritual nature. And because its quintessence is interconnectedness, transcending to the dimension of Atman means there is no you as a separate entity, no me as a separate entity. There is only spiritual universality. Atman is all selves.

Your knowledge and reverence of a divine place in you is where the proof of Atman lies. In other words, you can sense Atman's impact on your life by what transpires in your heart and how you act in the outer world. I am not referring to yogic method or ritual here. There is no yogic practice to access Atman because it isn't a kosha. The methods you've learned in this book will help lead you to your true essence, but Atman is not an experience to be had. It's the enlightenment of true self that lies at the beginning, end, and center of the kosha layers.

The sensation that comes from being divinely connected to your true essence can only be described in esoteric terms: You feel as if you've come home, and also there's a feeling of being at home in the presence of Atman. It's like a sigh of relief. You are beyond your ego—beyond your physicality, prana, thoughts, emotions, and inner wisdom. There's a deep bliss that transcends mere happiness or pleasure.

Your first glimmer of Atman may have occurred when you were working through chapter 5, on profound inner peace. As I explained in that chapter, the fifth kosha, or bliss body, closely surrounds your true essence. While profound inner peace is the subtlest of the koshas, it doesn't completely transcend who you are on a physical or perceptible plane. Atman does. How you choose to bridge Atman to your life in the material world—also known as the sixth kosha—is a significant indication of your own true transcendence.

THE SIXTH KOSHA—LOOKING OUTWARD

So far in this book, you've focused on deeper and deeper introspection, moving from the physical kosha layer to more inward and subtle layers of your being. Pull back from that internal perspective, though, and the sixth kosha comes into focus. The sixth kosha encompasses everything from the physical body outward. Basically, it's the external world in which you live.

In order to function optimally in the sixth kosha, you need to have a healthy relationship with your five internal koshas. When you lack a meaningful connection to your inner layers, you're at risk for defining yourself mostly by what happens in the sixth kosha, the outside world. For example, you might buy into advertising designed to push your emotional buttons, fear-based news reporting, office politics, or propaganda. Simply put, you may be more easily swayed or affected by external circumstances and stimuli. The ego world—meaning the people, things, and situations around you—may determine your destiny, level of happiness, and level of emotional pain. You will be less grounded in your understanding of your true self, which can cause you to lose control over your actions, reactions, and self-perceptions.

On the other hand, healthy connections to your inner koshas naturally foster a stronger sense of self and Atman. Through these connections, you become empowered to shift your outward perception so it stays true to your inner life. The benefits include more positive energy and greater love, kindness, and compassion for self and others. You will also begin to recognize Atman in all sentient beings. At this point, it makes sense to consider how you could manifest these meaningful inward experiences in transformative outward expressions.

INTEGRATING ATMAN INTO MODERN LIFE

I wrote this book as a blueprint for assimilating the ancient yogic philosophy of koshas into a modern era. The yoga methods in chapters 1 through 5 helped you explore the concept of nonattachment as you began to open yourself to the bliss of living from within, and living in the present. In chapter 4, on awareness, I mentioned that the outcomes of your intentions aren't as important as the process of acting on your intentions. The same concept of nonattachment applies here.

When you come from a place of nonattachment, you consciously pursue what feels right and joyous. Your life's vocation and other pursuits become an expression of your true essence. You choose your path as opposed to feeling obligated to fulfill the hopes and expectations of others at the expense of your personal joy. An example would be a musician who makes music for its own sake, not to be admired, strike it rich, or achieve success according to social standards. In the context of Atman, success—or lack of it—is circumstantial. The joy of expressing Atman is pure, so you do whatever it is that you do out of self-love, not to get something.

You might be wondering how you could survive in the world, pay your bills, take care of your family, and all the rest of it if you were to drop everything to satisfy your deepest joy, whatever that might be. Reverence to Atman isn't an expression of self-centeredness with no regard for others.

Sometimes—perhaps most of the time for most people—it's not realistic to begin a new life, and you might not want to anyway. What I am here to suggest, though, is that when you live joyfully in whatever capacity you are able, your bliss resonates in the universe and with those around you. You might have heard stories about people who started moonlighting, perhaps as an entertainer or caterer or educator, and their side business ended up becoming wildly profitable. I like to think this happens because of a subconscious resonance that occurs when people live out what pleases them most.

Even if you experience challenges along the way, having a rich connection to your inner koshas and Atman helps you process those difficulties as simply external bits of information, not bad luck, lack of talent, or something inherently hopeless about you. In other words, knowing your true essence provides a big-picture perspective so that you can comfortably handle the highs and lows you encounter in the external world.

PRACTICE KARMA YOGA

By this point, hopefully you've become personally familiar with the power of the five internal koshas. When your koshas are clarified, your true essence begins to shine more brightly. You start to inspire yourself from within. However, the internal work you've done so far is only half of the equation. The other half of this journey is applying what has surfaced in the external world. That might mean how you do your job, raise your kids, communicate with others, help people, give of yourself, contribute to your community, express your unique gifts and talents, and on and on. The ultimate goal is to express Atman in every moment of your life—or as much as possible. How you do that in the context of the sixth kosha, your outer reality, is self-defined and entirely up to you. I encourage you, however, to look beyond yourself toward the people and web of life around you. Consider how you can make a positive impact in the world. Preserve and build upon your blissfulness by serving others.

The simplest way to bridge your inner life to the outer world is through karma yoga, which is the expression of Atman in action. Previous chapters dealt with yoga for the bodily and internal realms. Karma yoga takes that internal enlightenment and radiates it outward. Think of karma yoga as a new enlightenment that makes a lot of sense in modern society. In ancient times, yogis would retreat from common life to connect more fully to Atman. That's not what you're here to do. Karma yoga is about consciously acting and living *within* the world around you.

The concept behind the Sanskrit word *karma* is that the effects of all deeds create your past, present, and future experiences. So putting goodness into the world brings goodness back to you. Being a karma yogi in life means contemplating and acting on how you can serve others. It's about giving, but also about accepting abundance on every level that it comes to you, including in a material sense. Living life to the fullest doesn't mean you'll make lots of money or are entitled to do so, nor does it mean renouncing wealth. Again, how you enjoy and act out your role as a karma yogi is purely self-defined. You might express karma yoga in traditional ways, such as by donating time or money to charities. But it doesn't have to start or end there. Karma yoga also consists of small deeds, such as opening a door for a stranger or smiling at people you encounter during your day. On a grander scale, you might practice karma yoga by trying to develop more intimacy and understanding in your relationships or by living your life's dream, or at least taking steps to get you there. Karma yoga is any deed, big or small, that spreads compassion, enjoyment, kindness, love, and understanding to the world. Here are some categories of good karmic deeds, and a few examples of each.

Environmental

- Help preserve and protect the planet by recycling more, turning off lights you don't need, using green products, and so on.

- Do your part to reduce pollution by walking or biking whenever possible instead of driving.

Interpersonal

- Seek to communicate with understanding and compassion with those around you.

- Focus on what others have to say; when appropriate, speak less and listen more.

Career

- Do your job to the best of your ability, and practice integrity in making career decisions.

- Seek balance in your life when it comes to how much time you spend working.

Creativity

- Pursue your creative passions, whether it's a hobby, a side business, an artistic endeavor, or your career.

- Share your creativity, talents, and passions with your family, friends, and coworkers, and with the world.

Charity

- Donate money, volunteer for a charitable organization, or give away material items you no longer need or want.

- Practice being charitable to others through compassion and respectfulness. Seek a greater understanding of the plights of others.

- Promote human welfare in large or small ways depending on the resources you possess.

Political Activism

- Stay informed about what's happening in your local and national government, as well as abroad.

- Voice your concerns to candidates and politicians, and make informed choices about who you vote for.

Spirituality

- Deepen your spirituality using the practices in this book, or any spiritual practice (such as prayer or spending time in nature) that feels like a good fit to you.

- Seek to understand how you are part of a greater whole, interconnected to all living beings.

To help you practice karma yoga, consider the following list of questions as food for thought:

- Do you aim to serve others?

- Are you coming from a place of joy?

- Are you acting in the best interest of both yourself and others?

- Do your actions inspire and uplift you and the people around you?

- Are your intentions aligned with your passions and principles?

- Are your actions leading you toward your goals and dreams?

- Do you foster intimacy and mutual respect in your relationships?

- Do you endeavor to create meaningful connections with others?

- Do you engage in spontaneous acts of kindness?

Answering yes to these questions helps you establish your own karma yoga rituals.

YOUR JOURNEY TOWARD UNLOCKING INNER BLISS

My hope is that the practices and concepts in this book will help you gain greater access to your inner koshas and true essence so you may live to your fullest potential in your day-to-day life in the real world. I leave you now with a reminder that the inward and outward yogic techniques in this book are meant to be part of an ongoing practice. While you might become quite skilled at some of the methods described here, there is no expected endpoint to your yoga practice. You could say that yoga is a lifelong companion. Think of it like eating breakfast, lunch, and dinner—naturally interwoven into your daily existence and, indeed, essential for your health and well-being. Nourish yourself with a consistent yoga "diet."

I encourage you to be patient in your exploration of the koshas. Remember the importance of non-attachment to outcome, and avoid worrying too much about achieving immediate or obvious results. Results will come, but the transformative part is the journey itself. Relish the process and the many life-affirming benefits of yogic living.

Also, be prepared for roadblocks and bumps along the way. At times in your life, you may go through hardship and challenges or feel doubt, fear, and a sense of imbalance. This doesn't negate the work you've done toward transformative yoga. In fact, it may signify that change is underway and that you're transcending toward a more joyful way of being, so don't feel discouraged.

I wish you all the best as you continue to explore the discipline of yoga and the wide world within you, and begin sharing the riches of your own budding bliss and enlightenment with the outer world around you.

APPENDIX:

POSTURE
CLASSIFICATIONS

Yoga postures can be defined according to a number of categories. Although the classifications below are based on physical position, they're also tied to the intention or benefits of the pose; for example, twists help promote spinal health and balance poses are especially good for activating your core muscles.

The lists below show how each posture in this book is classified and what some major benefits of those classifications are. You'll notice that basic poses often fall into just one category, while more advanced and complex postures might fit in multiple categories if the pose has more than one key intention.

SEATED

Benefits: Grounding, meditative
Beginner Accomplished Pose
Full Lotus
Half Lotus
Hero
Intermediate Accomplished Pose
Seated Cross-Legged
Seated Hand to Big Toe
Seated Legs Up and Apart
Seated L-Shaped Side Bend

SUPINE

Benefits: Relaxing, restorative, calming to the nervous system
    Both-Legs-Up Recline
    Knees to Chest
    Modified Happy Baby
    Relaxation Pose
    Supine Flexion
    Supine Straight Legs to Side

FORWARD BENDING

Benefits: Calming, relieves back tension, alleviates anxiety or worry
    Cat
    Child's Pose
    Knees to Chest
    One-Leg-Down Shoulder Stand
    Pigeon
    Plow
    Seated Legs-Apart Forward Bend
    Seated L-Shaped Forward Bend
    Standing Forward Bend
    Supine Flexion
    Wide-Leg Forward Bend

BACKWARD BENDING

Benefits: Stretches the chest, shoulders, or back of the body, strengthens and aligns the spine, counteracts low vitality and depression, opens the chest, invigorates
    Backbend Pigeon
    Bridge
    Camel
    Cow
    Dancer
    Exalted Warrior
    Extended Mountain
    Flag
    Full Wheel
    Gazing Halfway Up
    Half-Moon Leg Bent
    Table
    Upward Dog

TWISTING

Benefits: Promotes spinal health, relieves back tension, stretches the torso, upper back, shoulders, or neck

  Knee-Down Twist
  Reverse Triangle
  Seated Twist
  Twisting Hero
  Twisting Side Lunge

BALANCING

Benefits: Balances the right and left sides of the brain, activates the core

  Flying Crow
  Forearm Balance
  Half-Moon Leg Bent
  Hand to Big Toe
  Long Staff
  One-Legged Downward Dog
  Seated Hand to Big Toe
  Seated Legs Up and Apart
  Side Crow
  Tree
  Warrior 3

STANDING

Benefits: Invigorates, improves strength, stamina, and stability

  Dancer
  Extended Mountain
  Goddess
  Mountain
  Reverse Triangle
  Side Lunge
  Triangle
  Warrior 1
  Warrior 2

INVERTED

Benefits: Restorative, rests the heart, alleviates headaches, flushes the internal organs

Downward Dog
Headstand
One-Leg-Down Shoulder Stand
One-Legged Downward Dog
Plow
Shoulder Stand

Wade Imre Morissette has studied yoga for more than seventeen years with many of the world's most influential yoga teachers, including Baba Hari Das, Sri K. Pattabhi Jois, Sri Sri Ravi Shankar, T.K.V. Desikachar, and the Krishnamacharya Lineage. He is also a recording artist with Nutone Music. Morissette teaches weekend and week-long retreats that combine music, yoga, meditation, transformation, and personal development. For more information about these events, please visit www. wadeimremorissette.com.

Foreword writer **Alanis Morissette** is a Grammy Award-winning recording artist whose albums have sold more than sixty million copies worldwide. She has also acted in several films, television shows, and theater productions, including *Dogma, Sex and the City,* and *The Vagina Monologues.* She lives in Los Angeles, CA.

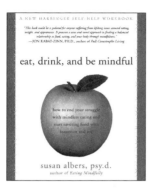
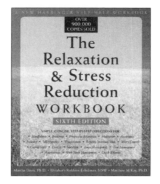
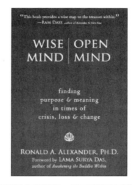
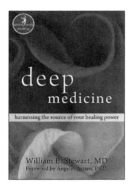
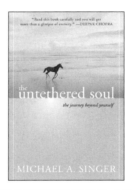
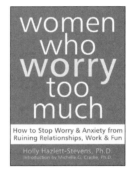